Monitoring for
Health Hazards at Work

Monitoring for Health Hazards at Work

Indira Ashton
BSc, MSc, PhD, MBA, MIOSH, MBIOH, DipSM, MSRP
Registered Safety Practitioner
Accredited Safety Auditor

Frank S. Gill
BSc, MSc, CEng, FBIOH, FFOM(Hon)., MAIOH
Consultant

Third Edition

Blackwell Science

© 1982, 1992, 2000 by
Blackwell Science Ltd

Editorial Offices:
Osney Mead, Oxford OX2 0EL
25 John Street, London
  WC1N 2BL
23 Ainslie Place, Edinburgh
  EH3 6AJ
350 Main Street, Malden
  MA 02148-5018, USA
54 University Street, Carlton
  Victoria 3053, Australia
10, rue Casimir Delavigne
  75006 Paris, France

Other Editorial Offices:
Blackwell Wissenschafts-Verlag
  GmbH, Kurfürstendamm 57
  10707 Berlin, Germany
Blackwell Science KK
  MG Kodenmacho Building
  7–10 Kodenmacho
  Nihombashi
  Chuo-ku, Tokyo 104, Japan

First Published 1982
Reprinted 1985
Second edition 1992
Third edition 2000

Set by Bookcraft Ltd, Stroud,
UK
Printed and bound in Great
Britain at the Alden Press Ltd,
Oxford and Northampton

The Blackwell Science logo is a
trade mark of Blackwell Science
Ltd, registered at the United
Kingdom Trade Marks Registry

A catalogue record for this title is
available from the British Library

ISBN 0-632-05041-1

Library of Congress Cataloging-
in-Publication Data

Ashton, Indira
    Monitoring for health hazards
    at work/
    Indira Ashton, Frank S. Gill.
    — 3rd ed.
        p.   cm.
    Includes bibliographical
    references and index.
    ISBN 0-632-05041-1
    1. Industrial toxicology.
    2. Environmental
    monitoring.
    I. Gill, F.S. (Frank S.)
    II. Title.
RA1229.A84 1999
615.9'02—dc21   99-32635
                            CIP

DISTRIBUTORS
Marston Book Services Ltd
PO Box 269
Abingdon, Oxon OX14 4YN
(*Orders*: Tel:. 01235 465500
          Fax:. 01235 465555)

USA
Blackwell Science, Inc.
Commerce Place
350 Main Street
Malden, MA 02148-5018
(*Orders*: Tel:. 800 759 6102
          . 781 388 8250
          Fax:. 781 388 8255)

Canada
Login Brothers Book
Company
324 Saulteaux Crescent
Winnipeg, Manitoba R3J 3T2
(*Orders*: Tel:. 204 837 2987)

Australia
Blackwell Science Pty Ltd
54 University Street
Carlton, Victoria 3053
(*Orders*: Tel:. 3 9347 0300
          Fax:. 3 9347 5001)

For further information on
Blackwell Science, visit our
website:
www.blackwell-science.com

Contents

List of Illustrations

List of Instruction Sheets

Preface

Since the introduction of the Health and Safety at Work (Etc.) Act, 1974, workplace environments and their related health hazards have come under closer scrutiny. Duties of employers under Section 2 of that Act require workplaces and the working environment to be 'safe and without risks to health ....' Since the publication of the first edition of this book a number of Regulations and Approved Codes of Practice made under the Health and Safety at Work (Etc.) Act, 1974 have been updated, notably in the areas of control of lead at work, work with asbestos insulation, radiological protection and asbestos coating. Several new Regulations with their associated Codes of Practice have been made, which include the Asbestos (Licensing) Regulations, 1983, the Asbestos (Prohibitions) Regulations, 1985, the Ionising Radiation Regulations, 1985, the Control of Substances Hazardous to Health Regulations, 1999 (COSHH), the Noise at Work Regulations, 1989, the Genetic Manipulation Regulations, 1990, the 'Six Pack' and others. The Act and its aftermath has therefore brought a greater awareness to employees that their place of work may be the cause of ill health and that their employers have a duty to safeguard health and ensure their comfort.

Since the enactment of this enabling legislation it has been necessary for management, often prompted by the workforce, to enquire into the possible health hazards present in the workplaces in their charge. Even places traditionally thought of as safe, such as offices, have experienced hazards associated with the introduction of new technology; and in manufacturing and service industries processes use chemicals and materials that are new and often inadequately tested for possible health risks. With the increased use of machinery, an increase in workplace hazards, including unacceptable noise levels and emission of heat and electromagnetic waves of various wavelengths and energies, became introduced. In addition, more detailed and intricate work requires better illumination and engineering controls. In order to assess the degree of risk to the workforce it is often necessary to measure the concentration or intensity of the suspected hazard, which may be airborne dust, gas, vapour, heat, noise, radiation or some other risk. It may also be necessary to review the reduction strategies of risk, the adequacy of control measures, and the performance of environmental control devices such as air conditioning, ventilation and lighting systems.

Although there is a body of people trained in the skills of workplace monitoring and control for health and comfort who practise under the name of 'occupational or industrial hygienists', at the time of writing there are fewer than 200 registered as Operational or Professional Hygienists in Great Britain. Many of these work for large companies or government bodies. Therefore the burden of finding someone competent to monitor a workplace falls on the shoulders of management who search within their companies for people with appropriate scientific training and experience to undertake this somewhat onerous task involving the use of instruments and equipment which require skill and insight to operate satisfactorily. People who often find themselves in this position are company chemists, safety officers, safety advisers, occupational health nurses, works engineers and others.

The Regulations and Codes of Practice which followed the 1974 Act have placed a duty on employers to keep an even keener watch on the environments in which their employees work. With regard to the COSHH and Noise Regulations, the number of fully and comprehensively trained occupational hygienists in the field has not significantly increased; therefore it is still necessary for company staff who have been trained initially in other disciplines to undertake monitoring for airborne substances and workplace noise. Furthermore, because of this recent legislation, the pressure to examine and monitor the working environment has increased.

The range of instruments and equipment available in the field is bewildering, and guidance on selection and use is required. Many of the monitoring and analysis techniques require the skills of analytical chemists, acousticians, ventilation engineers, microbiologists and health physicists, but workplace sampling and simple monitoring can be done by less-qualified 'in house' staff.

The purpose of this book is to provide guidance to personnel employed as safety and health professionals who have some responsibility for the protection of employees against health hazards at work and to those concerned with the planning and management of acceptable monitoring programmes and advising on control measures required. Also it is hoped that safety representatives and shop stewards will consult it to assist them to understand and, in some cases, advise management on risk assessment, minimisation of risk and methods of workplace measurement and sampling.

The book is written around a series of instruction sheets covering a variety of sampling and monitoring procedures grouped in suitable chapters. By way of introduction to the sheets a review of the types of instruments and equipment to be used is made, and some of the basic principles of the techniques and the factors to be taken into account when selecting instrumentation are described. Check lists are offered to assist in the assembly of items for a survey on a particular topic and, where appropriate, a method of recording the results is recommended. Lists of suppliers of equipment are also given together with their addresses. The instruction sheets and lists have been reviewed and updated during the preparation of this edition.

However, it is important to realise that there is no short cut to a full understanding of the science and behaviour of workplace hazards and pollution. The techniques described provide only an indication of the degree of hazard that is present. It must also be understood that workplace pollution of whatever kind is not evenly distributed in time or space; one single reading or measurement will not represent the workplace as a whole. Therefore, if major decisions are to be made based upon workplace environmental measurement then the best possible professional advice must be sought to plan and execute detailed surveys. The results can be confidently used to provide sound judgement on their meaning and to suggest the best course of action. The British Institute of Occupational Hygienists publishes a list of qualified consultants.

Readers are reminded that some workplace environments are contaminated with inflammable gases, vapours and dusts and that electrical equipment within them is required to be flameproof. This requirement extends to items of monitoring or sampling equipment both permanent and portable. Instruments that have been passed as suitable for use in such environments are issued with a British Approvals Service for Electrical Equipment in Flammable Atmospheres (BASEEFA) Certificate and care must be taken to ensure that only these are used. In case of doubt the manufacturer should be consulted.

It is good business sense and it is now built into statutory requirements that employers must aim to ensure that the health of employees and others is not damaged at work. Risk assessment is the essential first stage of any strategy to achieve this objective. Until an adequate analysis of a work area is carried out, it is not possible to set priorities for action and remedy any potential problems. Further, any solutions that are put into place may be ineffective and impractical. In this edition, a chapter on Assessment of risks to health has been included.

Publisher's note

Whilst the advice and information contained in this book are believed to be true and accurate at the date of going to press, neither the authors nor the publisher can accept any legal responsibility or liability for any errors or omissions that may have been made.

Acknowledgements

The authors would like to thank the many companies who have provided photographs and advice on their products.

The authors would also like to thank their families and friends who have given them support during the preparation of the book.

Units and Abbreviations*

The more common units used in workplace environmental measurement

Unit	Dimension	SI	Imperial	Conversion
Length	L	m	ft	$ft \times 0.3048 = m$
		mm	in	$in \times 25.4 = mm$
Area	L^2	m^2	ft^2	$ft^2 \times 9.29 \times 10^{-2} = m^2$
		mm^2	in^2	$in^2 \times 645.2 = mm^2$
Volume	L^3	m^3 (1000 litre)	ft^3	$ft^3 \times 2.832 \times 10^{-2} = m^3$
		l (litre)	gallon	$gallon \times 4.546 = litre$
Mass	M	kg	lb	$lb \times 0.4536 = kg$
		g (gram)	oz	$oz \times 28.35 = g$
		mg	grain	$gr \times 64.79 = mg$
Airborne concentration of substance				
(Mass)	$\dfrac{M}{L^3}$	$mg\ m^{-3}$	$grain\ ft^{-3}$	$gr\ ft^{-3} \times 2288 = mg\ m^{-3}$
(Volume)	—	—	parts per million (ppm)	
(Particle)	—	$mp\ cm^{-3}$	$mp\ ft^{-3}$	(millions of particles per cm^3 (ft^3))
Acceleration	$\dfrac{L}{T^2}$	$m\ s^{-2}$ gravity = 9.81 m s^{-2}	$ft\ sec^{-2}$	$ft\ s^{-2} \times 0.305 = m\ s^{-2}$
Density	$\dfrac{M}{L^3}$	$kg\ m^{-3}\ (g\ l^{-1})$	$lb\ ft^{-3}$	$lb\ ft^{-3} \times 16.02 = kg\ m^{-3}$
Flow rate				
(Mass)	$\dfrac{M}{T}$	$kg\ s^{-1}$	$lb\ hr^{-1}$	$lb\ hr^{-1} \times 1.26 \times 10^{-4} = kg\ s^{-1}$
(Volume)	$\dfrac{L^3}{T}$	$m^3\ s^{-1}$	$ft^{-3}\ min^{-1}$	$ft^3\ min^{-1} \times 4.719 \times 10^{-4} = m^3\ s^{-1}$
			$gall\ hr^{-1}$	$gall\ hr^{-1} \times 1.263 \times 10^{-6} = m^3\ s^{-1}$
Force	$\dfrac{ML}{T^2}$	N (Newton) (N = kg m s^{-2})	lb_f	$lb_f \times 4.448 = N$
Energy/ Heat quantity	$\dfrac{ML^2}{T^2}$	J (Joule) Ws = Nm kW hour	Btu	$Btu \times 1055 = J$ $kW\ hour \times 3.6 \times 10^6 = J$ $kilocalorie \times 4187 = J$
Heat flow/ Power	$\dfrac{ML^2}{T^3}$	W	HP $Btu\ hr^{-1}$	$HP \times 745.7 = W$ $Btu\ hr^{-1} \times 0.291 = W$
Latent heat	$\dfrac{L^2}{T^2}$	$kJ\ kg^{-1}$	$Btu\ lb^{-1}$	$Btu\ lb^{-1} \times 2.326 = kJ\ kg^{-1}$
Specific heat	$\dfrac{L}{T^2\ temp}$	$kJ\ kg^{-1}\ {}^\circ C$	$Btu\ lb^{-1}\ {}^\circ F$	$Btu\ lb^{-1}\ {}^\circ F \times 4.187 = kJ\ kg^{-1}\ {}^\circ C$

* In this book SI units are used throughout; however, conversions from Imperial to SI are given in the list of common units.

Unit	Dimension	SI	Imperial	Conversion
Pressure	$\dfrac{M}{T^2L}$	Pa (Pascal) = N m^{-2} bar ($\times 10^5$ = Pa)	lb$_f$ ft^{-2} lb$_f$ in^{-2} in water (4 °C) in mercury (0 °C)	lb ft^{-2} × 47.88 = Pa lb in^{-2} × 6895 = Pa in H$_2$O × 249.1 = Pa in Hg × 3386 = Pa
Torque	$\dfrac{ML^2}{T^2}$	Nm	lb$_f$ ft	lb$_f$ ft × 1.356 = Nm
Velocity	$\dfrac{L}{T}$	m s^{-1}	ft min^{-1} ft s^{-1}	ft m^{-1} × 5.08 × 10^{-3} = m s^{-1} ft s^{-1} × 0.305 = m s^{-1}
Viscosity				
(Dynamic)	$\dfrac{M}{TL}$	Pa s (Ns m^{-2}) Poise (dyne s cm^{-2})	lb.s ft^{-1}	lb.s ft^{-1} × 47.88 = Pa s Poise × 0.1=Pa s
(Kinematic)	$\dfrac{L^2}{T}$	m^2 s^{-1} Stokes (cm^2 s^{-1})	ft^2 s^{-1} in^2 s^{-1}	ft^2 s^{-1} × 9.29 × 10^{-2} = m^2 s^{-1} in^2 s^{-1} × 6.452 × 10^{-4} = m^2 s^{-1} Stokes × 10^{-4} = m^2 s^{-1}
Luminous intensity		candela (Cd)	candle (int)	candle × 0.981 = Cd
Luminous flux		lumen (1m) (lm = lCd sr)		
Illuminance		lux (lx = lm m^{-2})	foot candle lumen ft^{-2}	ft candle × 0.1076 = lx lm ft^{-2} × 0.1076 = lx
Luminance		Cd m^{-2}	foot lambert candela in^{-2}	ft lambert × 3.426 = Cd m^{-2} Cd in^{-2} × 1550 = Cd m^2
Radiation activity	dis s^{-1}	Bq	Ci	1 Ci = 3.1 × 10^{10} Bq = 3.7 × 10^4 MBq = 0.037 TBq 1 mCi = 37 × 10^6 Bq = 37 MBq = 3.7 × 10^{-5} TBq 1 µCi = 37 000 Bq = 0.037 MBq = 3.7 × 10^{-8} TBq 1 Bq = 2.7 × 10^{-5} µCi = 2.7 × 10^{-8} mCi = 2.7 × 10^{11} Ci 1 MBq = 27 µCi = 0.027 mCi = 2.7 × 10^{-5} Ci 1 TBq = 2.7 × 10^7 11Ci = 2.7 × 10^4 mCi = 27 Ci
Radiation absorbed dose	$\dfrac{J}{kg}$ kg	Gy	rad	1 Gy = 1 J kg^{-1} = 100 rad 1 mGy = 100 mrad 1 µGy = 0.1 mrad
Dose equivalent	rad × Q × N	Sv	rem	1 Sv = 100 rem 1 mSv = 100 mrem 1 µSv = 0.1 mrem

Temperature	° Celsius	° Fahrenheit	°F = (°C × 1.8) + 32
	−40	−40	
	−30	−22	
	−20	−4	
	−10	14	
	0	32	
	10	50	
	20	68	
	30	86	
	40	104	
	50	122	
	60	140	
	70	158	
	80	176	
	90	194	
	100	212	

Some useful initials

ACDP	Advisory Committee on Dangerous Pathogens
ACGIH	American Conference of Government Industrial Hygienists
ACOP	Approved Code of Practice
ACTS	Advisory Committee on Toxic Substances
ALARP	As low as reasonably practicable
ANSI	American National Standards Institute
BASEEFA	British Approvals Service for Electrical Equipment in Flammable Atmospheres
BIOH	British Institute of Occupational Hygienists
BOHS	British Occupational Hygiene Society (UK)
CAS	Chemical Abstract Series
CAWR	Control of Asbestos at Work Regulations
CEN	Comité Européan de Normalisation
CHIP	Chemicals (Hazard Information and Packaging for Supply Regulations)
CIBSE	Chartered Institute of Building Services Engineers
CIMAII	Control of Major Hazards Regulations
CLAW	Control of Lead at Work Regulations
COSHH	Control of Substances Hazardous to Health Regulations, 1998
DSE	Display screen equipment
EH	Environmental hygiene
EINECS	European Inventory of Existing Commercial chemical Substances
EMAS	Employment Medical Advisory Service (UK)
ERM	European Reference Method
HASAWA	Health and Safety at Work Etc. Act, 1974 (UK)
HSC	Health and Safety Commission (UK)
HSE	Health and Safety Executive (UK)
ICRP	International Commission on Radiological Protection
IES	Illuminating Engineering Society
ILO	International Labour Office
INIRC	International Non-Ionising Radiation Commission

IOM	Institute of Occupational Medicine
IRR	Ionising Radiation Regulations
ISO	International Organisation for Standardisation
MDHS	Methods of determining hazardous substances in air
MEL	Maximum exposure limit
MHSWR	Management of Health and Safety at Work Regulations
MRC	Medical Research Council (UK)
NIOSH	National Institute of Occupational Safety and Health (USA)
NPL	National Physical Laboratory
NRPB	National Radiological Protection Board
OEL	Occupational exposure limit
OES	Occupational exposure standard
OSHA	Occupational Safety and Health Administration
PPE	Personal protective equipment
PSPS	Pesticides Safety Precautions Scheme (UK)
RPA	Radiation Protection Adviser
RPE	Respiratory protective equipment
SI	Système International (International System of Units)
STEL	Short-term exposure limit
TWA	Time-weighted average
WATCH	Working Group on the Assessment of Toxic Substances
WHO	World Health Organisation
WRULD	Work-related upper limb disorder

Abbreviations in the text

Å	Ångstrom units
Bq	Becquerel
Btu	British thermal unit
Ci	Curie
°C	degree Celsius or centigrade
cd	candela
cfu	colony forming units
cm	centimetre
D	diameter
d	diameter or density correction factor
dB	decibel
E	illuminance
f	number of fibres
ft	foot
g	gram
g	acceleration due to gravity
gall	gallon
gr	grain
Gy	Gray
h	hour
Hg	mercury
Hz	hertz (cycles per second)
l	luminous intensity
in	inch
J	Joule
L	luminance or length
l	litre
lb	pound

lb$_f$	pound force
lm	lumen
lx	lux
M	mass
m	metre
mb	millibar
mCi	millicurie
mg	milligram
min	minute
mp cm^3	millions of particles per cubic centimetre
mp ft^{-3}	millions of particles per cubic foot
N	Newton or number of air changes per hour
oz	ounce
p	pressure
Pa	Pascal
ppm	parts per million
Q	quality factor
R	reflectance
rad	radiation absorbed dose
s	second
sr	steradian
rem	radiation dose equivalent
Sv	Sievert
t	time or temperature °C
T	absolute temperature (Kelvin) or time
V	volume or volume flow
v	velocity
W	Watt
μg	microgram
μm	micrometre
θ	Kata thermometer range
Φ	luminous flux
ρ	density
Δ	delta, meaning 'change of'

Multiples of SI units

Name	Symbol	Factor
tera	T	10^{12}
giga	G	10^{9}
mega	M	10^{6}
kilo	k	10^{3}
hecto	h	10^{2}
deca	da	10^{1}
deci	d	10^{-1}
centi	c	10^{-2}
milli	m	10^{-3}
micro	μ	10^{-6}
nano	n	10^{-9}
pico	p	10^{-12}
femto	f	10^{-15}
atto	a	10^{-18}

1 Dust

Introduction

Airborne dust is ubiquitous and workplaces are no exception; every operation and action releases a certain amount of dust into the air. Movement of people can release dust from clothing and skin. Even dust that has settled on floors and upper surfaces is made airborne by air currents as people move about their work. Windborne dust enters buildings particularly in dry weather and more so in densely populated areas. Add to that particles released by the operations within a workplace – handling and transfer of materials, machining, cutting, drilling, grinding, milling, sanding and planing of items being manufactured – and a dusty working atmosphere can be produced. Fortunately most dust is harmless but in sufficient concentrations it can cause discomfort and unpleasantness. At such levels it is termed a 'nuisance dust'. However, some dusts are distinctly harmful, giving rise to carcinoma, chronic lung disease, asthma, bronchitis and other disorders. A suspension of particles in air is referred to as an 'aerosol'.

Not only does the chemical composition of the material and its airborne concentration determine its detrimental effects but also the particle size influences the part of the lungs where the material is deposited. Large particles are collected in the nose and throat whilst smaller ones are deposited further into the lung, the next stage of collection being in the upper airways, i.e. the bronchi and bronchioles, where self-clearing action by the ciliary movement takes place. The very small particles reach the deepest parts, the alveoli, where the oxygen transfer takes place. Some particles are breathed out again and some are removed by body fluids but others remain and may cause physical and chemical reactions that can be harmful in both the short and long term, sometimes leading to permanent lung damage.

Dust size is measured in the unit called a micrometre (μm) which is a 1000th part of a millimetre; a human hair is above 30 μm in diameter. Unfortunately most particles of dust are irregular in shape and rarely spherical or circular, therefore it is difficult to quote size. The important feature is how dust behaves when it is airborne, particularly how rapidly it settles in still air. In the field of occupational health the term 'aerodynamic diameter' is used to denote the particles' size. This is the diameter of a theoretical spherical particle of unit density (1 g ml^{-1}) which settles at the same speed as the particle in question; thus any irregularly shaped particle can be assigned an aerodynamic diameter. Dust that can be

1

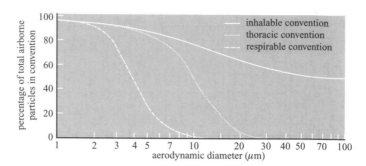

Fig. 1.1. ISO/CEN/ACGIH sampling conventions for health-related aerosols.

inhaled reaches different parts of the lung, depending upon its aerodynamic diameter. Collaboration between three international organisations, ISO, CEN and ACGIH, has produced agreement on the definition of health-related aerosol fractions. The sizes are termed *inhalable* fraction, *thoracic* fraction and *respirable* fraction, and are best defined by means of a graph shown in Fig. 1.1.

• The inhalable fraction, which includes the thoracic and respirable fractions, is defined as the mass fraction of total airborne particles that are inhaled through the nose and/or mouth.

• The thoracic fraction, which includes respirable fraction, is defined as the mass fraction that penetrates the respiratory system beyond the larynx.

• The respirable fraction is defined as the mass fraction that penetrates to the unciliated airways of the lung, known as the alveolar region, where the gas exchange takes place. It is represented by a cumulative log-normal curve having a median aerodynamic diameter of 4.25 μm and a standard deviation of 1.5. From the curve in Fig. 1.1 it can be seen that dust particles larger than 10 μm cannot reach this region of the lung.

Dust from coal, sand and most hard rocks is harmful at respirable/alveolar size but is normally cleared from the lung if larger; whereas pollens, spores and mists are larger but 'inspirable' and can cause problems in the upper respiratory passages. Fumes from vaporised metal contain particles that are very small, below 1 μm, and can give rise to metal fume fever and more serious disorders. When determining the concentration of airborne dust it is important to understand what size of dust is to be measured as this influences the method of sampling.

Fibres

Fibres are a special type of particle that are longer than their width by a ratio of 3:1 (known as aspect ratio). Their aerodynamic diameters bear little relationship to either their width or length. They form an important group of particles as they include highly toxic material such as asbestos, which lead to serious lung damage at respirable sizes. They can be classified into four groups: natural vegetable, natural mineral, man-made organic and man-made mineral, as described below.

Natural vegetable – from plants and include: cotton, hemp, jute, sisal, i.e. the natural constituents of textiles.

Natural mineral – from the earth's crust, consisting of various types of asbestos occurring as crystals that are much longer than their width and have great strength and excellent fire-resistance and thermal-insulation properties. They are subdivided into two mineral groups: serpentines (hydrated magnesium silicate) and amphiboles (calcium, magnesium, sodium and iron silicates). The serpentines have only one fibrous form, known as chrysotile (white asbestos): when an airborne sample is viewed under a microscope most fibres appear to have a curly shape. The amphiboles have several fibrous forms: crocidolite (blue asbestos), amosite, tremolite and anthophyllite. When airborne samples are viewed under a microscope they appear to have straight, needle-like fibres, although more elaborate techniques are required to positively identify the fibre type. Asbestos fibres less than 3 μm in diameter are respirable – that is, they will reach the gas-exchange parts of the lungs known as alveoli where they may cause damage – but it is thought that the amphiboles are more toxic than the serpentine. Methods of sampling for airborne asbestos fibres are described later in this chapter.

Man-made organic – these appear as trade names such as nylon, orlon, crimplene and rayon, and are mainly used in the textile industry. They are always larger in diameter than 3 μm.

Man-made mineral – mainly used as a replacement for asbestos in thermal insulation and made of a variety of substances such as glass, rock, carbon/graphite, aromatic diamines and polyolefines. Most of these fibres are larger in diameter than 3 μm but a few can be below this size and may be regarded as toxic.

The Health and Safety Executive (HSE) publish guidance on sampling for airborne asbestos and airborne man-made mineral fibres in their series, Methods of Determining Hazardous Substances (MDHS).

Sampling for airborne dust

There are two basic methods of sampling airborne dust: (a) filtration sampling; and (b) use of direct-reading instruments.

The first, and most common, is to draw a known volume of air through a pre-weighed filtering device by means of an air pump. Weighing the filtering device before and after will determine the mass of dust collected. By dividing that mass by the total volume of air drawn through, an average dust concentration is obtained for the sampling period.

The second method involves using an instrument that gives a direct reading of the dust concentration at any instant of time but may or may not give an average over a period of time.

Filtration systems are available that are lightweight enough for employees to wear to determine their personal exposure to the airborne dust. If they move about in and out of dust clouds or if the emission varies in concentration the readings monitor the average exposure.

The filtration method can also be used to monitor a working area using one static position throughout the sampling period. In this case the equipment should, if possible, be attached to a tripod or fixed object in the area under study. In order to achieve sufficient accuracy it is important to weigh the filters to 0.01 mg. Since this may be beyond the precision of most laboratory balances it requires a micro-analytical balance capable of weighing to 1 μg. Also the flow rates of the pumps must be checked with a calibrated rotameter so that the total flow rate passing through the filter is accurately known. A section on calibrating a rotameter is included below (see page 13).

The direct reading instruments are more bulky and are unsuited to personal monitoring; they are used to measure a working area rather than an individual. A review of some of these instruments is given later (see page 12).

Equipment required for filtration sampling

An assembly of items is required to make up a sampling 'train' consisting of:
1 An appropriate filter.
2 An appropriate filter holder.
3 A suction pump.
4 Some connecting tubing.
5 A harness.

In addition a rotameter or flowmeter is required to check air-flow rates.

Filters

These are made of a variety of materials with properties suited to different types of analyses. This is covered in more detail below (see page 31). Filters are mainly 'fibrous' in structure, made from glass, paper, polystyrene or from a 'membrane' of cellulose derivatives, PVC and polycarbonate. There is also a sintered silver filter available. The correct filter must be chosen to suit the airborne contaminant to be sampled and the subsequent analysis to be undertaken; for example, some can be dissolved in chemicals for further analysis of the collected dust, some can be made transparent for optical microscopic examination of the material, whilst others allow the collected dust to remain on the surface for scanning electron microscopic examination. Some filters are more sensitive to atmospheric moisture content than others, and need to be pre-conditioned before weighing.

Filters used for dust sampling are available in diameters of 13, 25, 37, 47, 50, 55 mm, and larger. The smaller filters are more commonly used for personal sampling and the larger ones for high-volume work. Pore sizes vary between 0.1 μm to 10 μm but it should be noted that the pore size does not limit the size of the dust to be collected; that is, a 5 μm pore size filter is capable of capturing dusts smaller than 5 μm by virtue of the inertial and electrostatic forces that occur within the filter medium. In fact it is often desirable to use pore sizes in the range 5–10 μm even for respirable dusts, to reduce the loading on the sampling pump. For particle and fibre counting with a light microscope it is useful to have the filter marked with a squared grid as it assists in focusing.

Filter holders

In order to accommodate the filter and to make a connection via tubing to the sampling pump a filter holder is required, which can be attached to a person as close to the nose as possible in an area known as the breathing zone. The holder usually has a clip so that it can be hung from a collar or from a harness, useful if the employee wears a T-shirt. Proprietory holders have buckles to allow snug fitting to whatever size of employee is to wear them. Figure 1.16 shows a harness being worn.

The filter holder is designed either to collect inhalable dust on the filter or to separate the respirable fraction, discarding anything larger than 10 μm. A special holder is also available for sampling asbestos and another for lead. A range of holders is available for inhalable dust as shown Figs 1.2 a, b and c. The seven-hole holder, Fig. 1.2a, has been in use for many years but now has two competitors, which make use of a filter cassette: the IOM holder, Fig. 1.2b, and the conical inhalable sampler, Fig. 1.2c. The first two take 25 mm diameter filter papers whilst the latter takes 37 mm

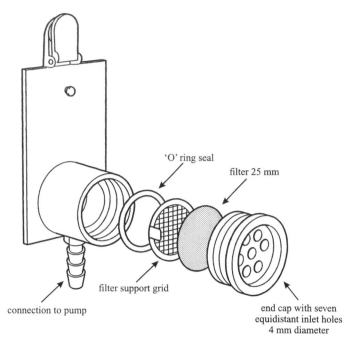

Fig. 1.2a. Multi-orifice total inhalable sampler (HSE).

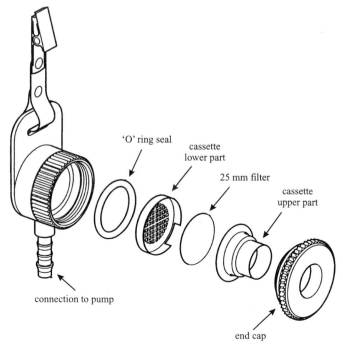

Fig. 1.2b. IOM inhalable sampler (HSE).

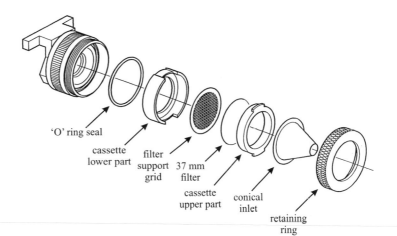

'O' ring seal

cassette
lower part

filter
support
grid

37 mm
filter

cassette
upper part

conical
inlet

retaining
ring

Fig. 1.2c. Conical inhalable sampler (HSE).

diameter papers. The advantage of using a cassette is ease of handling and fewer damaged or contaminated filters; the filter is protected once it has been weighed in the cassette, and can be transported within the cassette and loaded into the holder without further handling.

For asbestos sampling the filter holder is of a type shown in Fig. 1.3, known as the ERM holder, which has a tubular cowl to protect the filter. Its use is recommended in HSE guidance EH10.

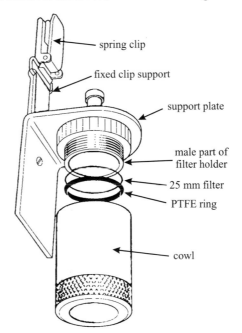

spring clip

fixed clip support

support plate

male part of
filter holder

25 mm filter

PTFE ring

cowl

Fig. 1.3. Cowled sampling head for asbestos and other fibres (HSE).

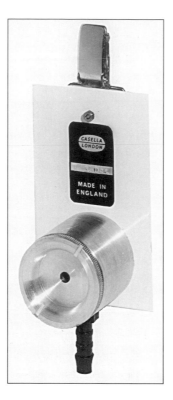

Fig. 1.4. Single-hole filter holder (Casella).

For lead, the holder has a single 4 mm diameter hole as shown in Fig. 1.4 and is recommended for use with lead in HSE guidance EH28. It is advisable to use the single-hole holder for heavy dusts such as mercuric oxide as it protects the filter from particles beyond total inhalable size that may be projected on to it. Since the mass of a particle is proportional to the cube of its diameter, one oversize particle will weigh many times more than an inhalable one and may give a falsely high result.

Respirable dust is sampled using a cyclone filter holder, which uses centrifugal force to separate dust particles larger than 10 μm. The dust-laden air spins within the cyclone allowing larger particles to be thrown to the outside of the holder and thence down into a pot at the base. The finer dust particles remain airborne and are collected on the filter. It is important to ensure the correct airflow rate to make the size cut-off follow the respirable curve in Fig. 1.1. The cyclone illustrated in Fig 1.5 achieves this by having a sampling flow rate of 2.2 1 min^{-1}.

For static sampling for respirable dusts some units have a combined pump and filter holder, for example the MRE 113 shown in Fig. 1.6. This was commonly used in mines in Great Britain. In this sampler, size selection for the respirable particles is achieved by means of an 'elutriator' where the larger sizes settle on to a series

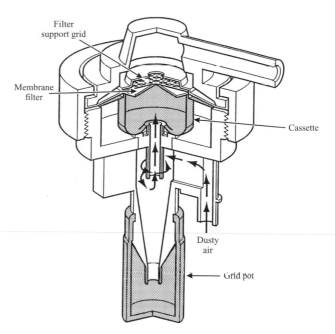

Fig. 1.5. Cyclone respirable sampler (HSE).

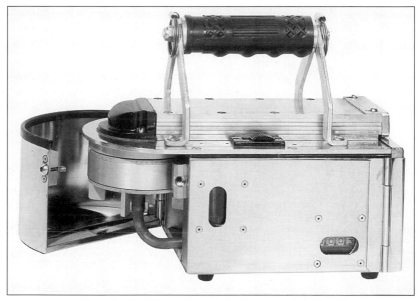

Fig. 1.6. MRE 113 static respirable dust sampler (Casella Ltd).

of parallel plates between which the dust-laden air passes before reaching the 55 mm diameter filter. As with all size-selection techniques the sampled air-flow rate must be fixed and constant for more accurate sampling.

Sampling pumps

There are three basic types of pump unit: the dry vane rotary, the single acting diaphragm used in the Casella, Dupont and MSA pumps (Fig. 1.8), and the double acting piston. Table 1.1 summarises the characteristics of each type. For dust sampling the rotary pumps produce the smoothest flow rates; the piston and diaphragm pumps produce a pulsating flow and require a flow 'smoother' to be added to the sampling train if particle size selection is being made. Most of the latest pumps have a flow smoother integral with the pump, and some have built-in rotameters but these may not be precise.

For personal sampling, easily portable battery operated pumps are used, some of which can achieve flow rates of up to 4.5 l min^{-1}. Some have rotameter-type flowmeters built in so that flow rates can be visibly checked from time to time, but some diaphragm pumps are fitted with a stroke counter to indicate the number of pulses of the diaphragm that have occurred during the sampling period and, from this, the total flow can be calculated. These medium flow pumps are battery powered using rechargeable batteries and the suppliers include chargers amongst their products. However, it is possible to fit disposable dry batteries to pumps and some occupational hygienists prefer this option as it removes the uncertainties concerning the state of charge of the rechargeable ones. That is, new dry batteries are fitted at the beginning of each sampling period and discarded at the end. Modern pumps have automatic constant flow control and some have timers to start and stop at pre-set times and to record the elapsed time.

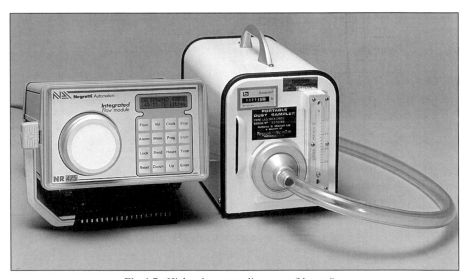

Fig. 1.7. High volume sampling pump (Negretti).

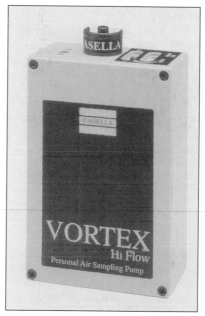

Fig. 1.8. Personal sampling pump (Casella).

To collect quantities of dust over a reasonable period of time that provide an adequate sample for subsequent weighing or other forms of analysis, fairly high flow rates may be required. This is normally easier to achieve for static sampling where mains powered pumps capable of up to 100 l min^{-1} are available.

Table 1.1. Characteristics of personal sampling pumps

Pump type	Diaphragm	Piston	Rotary
Power consumption	Low	Medium	High
Battery size	Small	Medium	Large
Weight	Low	Medium	High
Repair	Simple	Difficult	Moderate
Cost	Cheap	High	Medium
Flow smoothness	Strongly pulsating one pulse per rev.	Mildly pulsating two pulses per rev.	Smooth, three or four pulses per rev.
Pressure drop limits	4.9 kPa	None	None
Valve problems*	Can leak	Can leak	None (no valves)
Manufacturer	Casella, DuPont, MSA	Pitman	Negretti

* It is advisable always to run a pump with a filter fitted to avoid particles of dust being drawn onto the valve seats or into the rotor, which can be damaged by the particles.

Direct reading instruments

Compared with the filter method, which requires calculations and the use of accurate weighing techniques, direct reading instruments have the advantage that localised peaks of concentration can be identified and remedial measures immediately put into effect. They can be coupled to a recording system to obtain time-weighted average concentrations and real-time exposures. Unfortunately, due to their bulk, it is almost impossible to obtain personal exposure measurements with them and their calibration is questionable, being dependent upon the type and size of the particles sampled. They are far more expensive to buy than the equipment required for the filtration methods.

For their operation the instruments rely upon one of the following physical principles: the scattering of light by airborne particles of dust; the beta-ray absorption of a deposit of dust on a mylar film, or the oscillation frequency variation of a crystal of quartz when laden with dust (this latter technique is known as a 'piezo-electric' microbalance). Most of the instruments have a digital display or a meter which gives a reading of dust concentration in mg m^{-3}. One make, the Royco, provides a particle count. Because of the variations of physical properties of dust the instruments cannot be accurate for all types so they require careful calibration with the dust to be measured with a known concentration. One make, the SIMSLIN (Fig. 1.9) incorporates a facility for collecting a sample of the dust that has passed through the

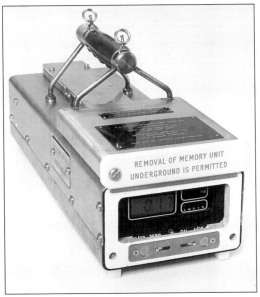

Fig. 1.9. SIMSLIN II direct reading dust sampler (Negretti Automation Ltd).

instrument on a membrane filter so that calibration can be achieved by comparing the average recorded dust concentration with that calculated from the weight gain of the filter.

As the number of direct reading instruments available is increasing and the design is continually being improved, it is advisable to discuss requirements with a technical representative from the suppliers (see Appendices I and II, Suppliers of equipment and Addresses of suppliers) before making a choice. Examples of direct reading dust monitors are shown in Figs 1.10–1.12.

Calibration of a rotameter using a soap bubble method

Aim
When sampling for dust or gases in a work situation, from time to time it is necessary to check the flow rate of air being drawn through the sampling train by the pump. A portable rotameter, which consists of a graduated tube containing a small float, is often used. The indicated flow rate is read from the graduation level with the top of the float. The rotameter must first be calibrated – the soap bubble technique is a cheap and reliable method for doing this.

Equipment required
A steady flow-rate sampling pump capable of supplying air at the flow rate of the rotameter to be calibrated, a glass burette graduated in millilitres, the rotameter to be calibrated, a rubber bulb, a glass T-piece, some flexible tubing of suitable size to connect the items, two stands, boss heads and clamps, tubing clips, liquid soap, cotton wool, stop-watch or timer, beaker. The size of the burette will depend upon the range of the rotameter to be calibrated; for medium-flow-rateflow-rate pumps, that is $1.0–4.5\ 1\ min^{-1}$, a burette of 250 ml capacity is most suitable but for lower flow rates a 100 ml size is sufficient.

Some pump manufacturers supply their own soap bubble calibrators which, although more expensive than assembling the equipment above, are self-contained and may be less trouble. An example is shown in Fig. 1.13.

Method
1   Wash the burette with water and then wet the inside surfaces with a thin film of the liquid soap. This can be done by pouring in a little of the soap and washing it down with water from a beaker.
2   Assemble the apparatus as shown in Fig. 1.14 and place a small plug of cotton wool at the top of the burette to prevent soap from being drawn into the pump.
3   Place some of the liquid soap in the rubber bulb.

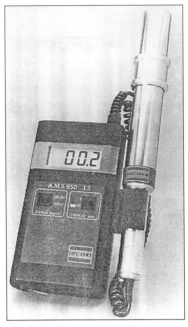

Fig. 1.10. Casella AMS950 hand-held aerosol monitor (Casella Ltd).

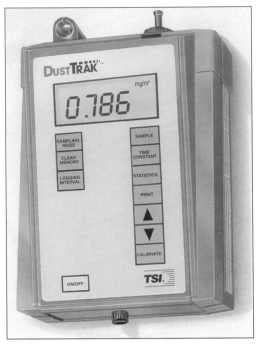

Fig. 1.11. TSI Dust Track™ respirable aerosol monitor (BIRAL).

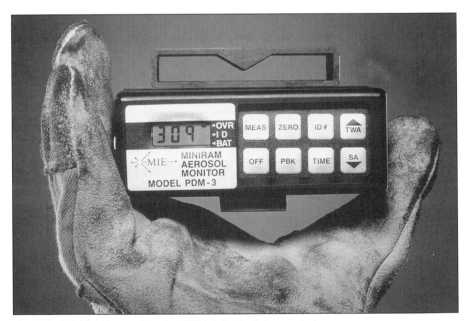

Fig. 1.12. Mini-RAM aerosol monitor PDM–3 (Analysis Automation).

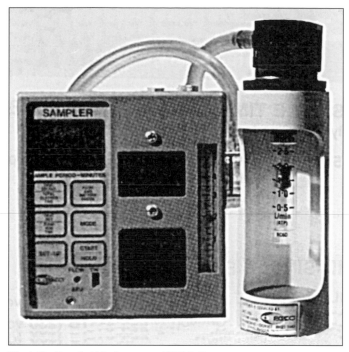

Fig. 1.13. Soap bubble flow meter (SKC Ltd).

4   Clamp the rotameter in a vertical position using the retort stand and fittings.
5   Start the pump to draw air through the system.
6   Squeeze the rubber bulb gently to release some soap into the airstream so that a bubble will be formed.
7   Time the bubble passing between the 0 and 250 ml marks on the burette and repeat this five times for one particular setting of the flow. When observing the position of the bubble for timing it is important to keep one's eye level with the mark.
8   By means of a tubing clamp or by altering the pump flow rate the position of the float in the rotameter can be altered and steps 6 and 7 can be repeated. This should be done for several flow rates throughout the range of the rotameter.

Results and calculations
Using a chart similar to Table 1.2 record or plot the results as they are taken.
To calculate actual flow, F_a, use the expression

$$F_a = \frac{V}{t} \times 60 \, \mathrm{l \, min^{-1}}$$

where V = the swept volume of the bubble in litres (1 litre = 1000 ml), and t = the mean time in seconds.

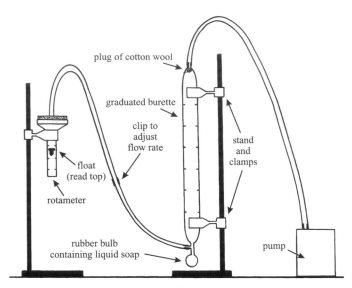

Fig. 1.14. Diagram of apparatus to calibrate a rotameter.

Plot the calculated mean flow rates against the rates marked on the stem of the rotameter as shown in the graph in Fig. 1.15. This graph should always be carried with the rotameter for checking the pump flow rates during surveys or tests.

Table 1.2.   Results sheet for the calibration of a rotameter

Indicated flow on rotameter ($l \, min^{-1}$)		0.5	1.0	1.5	2.0	2.5	3.0	3.5	4.0
Time taken for bubble to travel between marks (s)	Readings: 1								
	2								
	3								
	4								
	5								
Mean of the five readings									
Actual flow ($l \, min^{-1}$)									

Possible problems

1   The rotameter float may be pulsating due to the pump having a pulsating flow characteristic. To reduce this, either fit a flow-smoother into the line or change to a rotating-vane pump.

2   The soap bubble may burst before reaching the end of its travel, due to the sides of the burette being too dry. The burette should be removed from its clamps and the sides wetted with liquid soap and water as in step 1 in the method section.

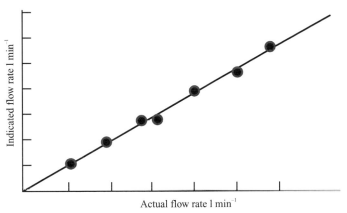

Fig. 1.15. Typical rotameter calibration chart.

The measurement of inhalable airborne dust

Aim

This, the most basic of airborne dust measuring techniques, is used to obtain a general total dust concentration in the breathing zone of an employee or in a particular static position. The technique is modified if a specific size range or type of dust is required to be collected and assessed. Such modifications involve changing the type of filter and/or filter holder as indicated in later sections of this chapter. It is normal to place the sampling head on the lapel of the operative. This may not be the most representative position since airborne particles can impinge on the filter from the process being undertaken and in so doing cause overestimation of the true inhaled concentration. If this occurs, then sampling closer to the nose is preferred. However, this involves making up a special head band to hold the apparatus. Alternatively, it could be attached to protective clothing worn on the head such a welder's visor.

Equipment required

For each place to be sampled simultaneously, a sampling pump capable of a flow rate of 1.0–4.5 l min^{-1}; a clean filter holder, seven-hole or Institute of Occupational Medicine (IOM) type, capable of holding a 25 mm diameter filter; one metre of 7 mm internal diameter plastic tubing; a calibrated rotameter (see above); 25 mm glass fibre filters; forceps; harness or head band to carry filter holder; a balance capable of weighing to 0.01 mg; labels; Petri-slides; and, if static samples are to be collected, then some form of substantial stand such as a heavy photographic tripod and some means of attaching the holder and pump to it such as adhesive tape or string is needed.

Method

1   Because the weight of filters tends to vary with the humidity of the air, it is wise to allow them to become pre-conditioned by placing each one in a Petri-slide to stand overnight in the room in which they are to be weighed.

2   Always handle filters with forceps and weigh the filters to 0.01 mg. Weigh more filters than are required for sampling so that one can be used as a control and the others are spares in case of accidental damage or contamination. If a filter is accidentally dropped or touched after weighing then it must be discarded as the weight will be altered. If an IOM holder is used, place the filter in the cassette and weigh.

3   Transport each of the weighed filters to the measuring site in a separate labelled Petri-slide or in a covered cassette.

4   Unscrew the front of the filter holder and using forceps or tweezers carefully place one weighed filter on the grid and replace the front. Do not over-tighten as the filters can easily be damaged. It is important to number and label each filter holder.

Note: it may be more convenient to place the filter in the holder immediately after weighing and transport it to the site in the holder suitably covered.

With the cassette type of filter holder, carefully remove the cover clip and place the cassette into the holder. Screw the cover down firmly but, to avoid damage to the holder, do not over-tighten.

5   Make up the sampling train by connecting the filter holder to the pump by means of the plastic tubing and place in the sampling position. If the measuring position is on an employee then it is best that the whole assembly is held in position by means of a harness (Fig. 1.16).

6   Attach the filter holder face forwards as close to the worker's face as possible on the front of the shoulder strap and hang the pump on the belt. If a static measuring position is to be taken, then attach the filter holder securely in place, preferably to a tripod.

7   Switch on the pump noting the time, and by means of the calibrated rotameter note the flow rate of air passing through the sampling train and adjust if necessary to the desired flow rate. To check the flow rate place the face of the filter holder tightly down on to the sponge seal of the rotameter and by holding the glass tube of the rotameter in a vertical position at eye level observe the position of the float as shown in Fig. 1.17. The mark level with the top of the float indicates the flow rate. It will be necessary to check the pump flow rate from time to time during the sampling period and adjust if necessary to attempt to maintain a constant flow rate. Some pump flow rates can be adjusted by turning a

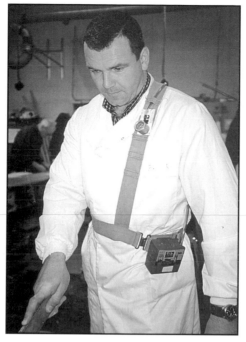

Fig. 1.16. Sampling train being worked on a harness with multi-orifice sampling head.

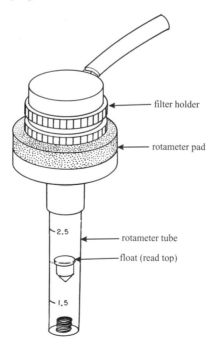

filter holder

rotameter pad

2.5

rotameter tube

float (read top)

1.5

Fig. 1.17. Rotameter in use with open face filter holder.

controlling screw by means of a small screwdriver, but others cannot be adjusted. Some pump designs have an automatic flow adjuster, which maintains a constant flow throughout the monitoring period. Some pumps have a pulse counter or a timer whose value must be noted at the beginning and end of the period. The length of time of sampling will depend upon circumstances, but precision will be lost if an insufficient volume of air is drawn through the filter. Recommended minimum sampling times from the volume should be calculated from the following expression:

$$\text{Minimum volume } (m^3) = \frac{10 \times \text{sensitivity of the balance (mg)}}{\text{suitable hygiene standard (mg m}^{-3})}$$

The suitable hygiene standard chosen will depend upon the dustiness of the place sampled but it is suggested that if this is in doubt then one-tenth of the occupational exposure standard should be used. Should it be necessary to stop and restart the pump at any time during the test then all times must be noted and flow rates checked.

8   At the end of the sampling period stop the pump and note the time.

9   After exposure carefully remove the filter using forceps and return it to the labelled Petri-slide, or remove the cassette.

10   A period of pre-conditioning in the balance room similar to that used for the initial weighing should elapse before re-weighing. The control filter should also be pre-conditioned and re-weighed.

11   Record all readings and results as they are made. A table similar to Table 1.3 can be used to record the results.

Calculations

Determine the total volume of air (V) that has passed through the filter using the expression:

$$V = \frac{\text{flow rate of pump in 1 min}^{-1} \times \text{duration in min}}{1000} \; m^3$$

Note: if the flow rate has changed during the period this calculation must be carried out for each change of rate and all the volumes added together.

To calculate the true weight gain of the filter proceed as follows:

wt. of filter before exposure	$= x_1 \, (mg)$
wt. of filter after exposure	$= x_2 \, (mg)$
wt. of control filter before	$= z_1 \, (mg)$
wt. of control filter after	$= z_2 \, (mg)$
wt. of dust on filter	$= x_2 - x_1 \left(z_2 - z_1 \right) (mg)$

Table 1.3. Suggested layout for a dust sampling results sheet

Survey . . . . Sampled by . . . .

Location . . . . Date . . . .

Filter no.	Pump no.	Sampling position	Sampling time			Flow rates		Total volume	Weight of filter	Weight of filter and dust	Weight gain	Dust concentration	Remarks
			On	Off	Total	Measured	Corr. av.						
					min	$l\,min^{-1}$	$l\,min^{-1}$	m^3	mg	mg	mg	$mg\,m^{-3}$	

$$\text{Concentration of dust in air in mg m}^3 = \frac{\text{wt. of dust on filter (mg)}}{V\,(\text{m}^3)}$$

Possible problems

1   Care must be taken to ensure that the filters are not contaminated either accidentally or deliberately by extraneous dust being allowed to come into contact with them. They must always be handled with forceps or tweezers. The single-hole type of filter holder should be used if there is a risk that large particles of dust, which are unlikely to be inhaled, could be projected towards the filter and should always be used when sampling for heavy dusts such as lead or compounds of lead or mercury.

2   If the pump flow rate change has not been noticed during the period, then an estimate can be made of the total flow based upon what flows have been noted, but the resulting calculations will be a rough estimate of the true dust concentration.

3   Damaged filters must be discarded and those samples discounted.

4   Filters can be overloaded if the sampling rate is too high or if the dust concentration is very dense. If this is suspected a lower flow rate or a shorter sampling period should be adopted.

5   Over-loaded filters can lose dust during handling and transport.

The measurement of airborne respirable dust using a cyclone separator

Aim

In order to separate the respirable or alveolar fraction of airborne dust from the total dust a modification of the basic open face filter method is adopted. The filter holder used is a cyclone separator, which, at a flow rate of $2.2\,\text{l min}^{-1}$, will separate dust according to the respirable curve in Fig. 1.1. The technique is similar to sampling for total or inhalable dust except that it is important to maintain a smooth flow rate at a steady $2.2\,\text{l min}^{-1}$ throughout the sampling period. For this purpose it is useful to make use of one of the controlled flow-rate pumps.

Equipment required

For each place to be sampled simultaneously, a cyclone separator and a pump capable of a smooth flow rate of at least $2.2\,\text{l min}^{-1}$. Pumps that operate on a rotary principle (see Table 1.1) provide a sufficiently steady flow rate for satisfactory separation but pumps with a reciprocating action require a flow smoothing device to ensure a smooth flow at the cyclone. The Higgins cyclone takes

25 mm diameter filters but the SIMPEDS cyclones take 37 mm unless fitted with a 25 mm cassette. The remaining equipment required is the same as for the measurement of total dust using an open face filter.

Method
1   Filters should be weighed in the same way as steps 1 and 2 on page 18.
2   Loading the filters into the cyclone varies with the type of separator used. With the Higgins cyclone it is necessary to dismantle the instrument and place the 25 mm filter on the grid (see Fig. 1.18), then carefully reassemble ensuring that the two halves of the cyclone are not over-tightened, to prevent the filter from becoming damaged. With the SIMPEDS cyclone the filter is assembled into a cassette held together by a wide elastic band (see Fig. 1.19). This is best done in a jig provided for the purpose. Adapters are available to enable a 25 mm filter to be placed in a 37 mm cyclone.
3   The sampling procedure is the same as for the open face filter, steps 5 to 11, except that the sampling rate must be maintained at 2.2 l min^{-1}, which should be checked regularly during the sampling period using a calibrated rotameter. The base of the Higgins cyclone can be held tightly against the sponge pad of the rotameter and the tube held vertically at eye level to read. With the SIMPEDS cyclone it is necessary to connect the rotameter to the inlet nozzle by means of tubing.

Calculations
These are exactly the same as with the open face filter method outlined on page 20.

Possible problems
1   If the pump flow rate has changed during the sampling period then the filter has not collected a representative sample of respirable dust, although a tolerance of 0.1 l min^{-1} above or below that can be accepted. If the flow rate has reduced then dust larger than respirable size will have been collected giving an exaggeratedly high result. The opposite would have occurred if the flow rate had been above 2.2 l min^{-1}.
2   The mass of a particle of dust varies with the cube of the diameter, and respirable dust is so small it will be very light in weight. Thus it is often difficult to obtain a sufficiently large weight gain on the filter to give a reliable result. To minimise this effect sampling durations should be as long as possible.
3   Damaged filters must be discarded as it is impossible to obtain a meaningful weight gain from them.

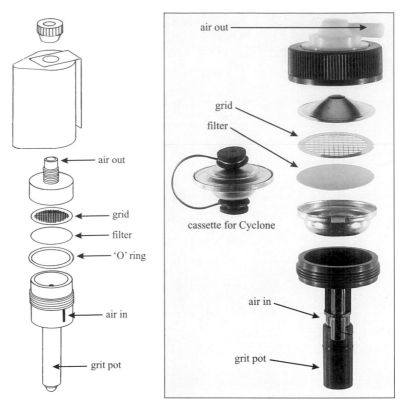

Fig. 1.18. *(left)* Exploded view of the Higgins cyclone.

Fig. 1.19. *(right)* Exploded view of the SIMPEDS cyclone (Casella Ltd).

4 In some workplaces dust is emitted in a concentrated stream and in a predictable direction. Care must then be taken to ensure that it is not projected directly on to the filter. It may be necessary to move the holder to a position out of the stream.

The sampling and counting of airborne asbestos fibres

Aim

Asbestos is present in many work situations, for example, as thermal insulation on pipes, building surfaces, vehicle linings; as an acoustic absorbent material on walls, ceilings, silencers; as a building material such as roofs, walls, pipes and gutters; in vehicle brake linings; and in many other places where its useful properties are utilised. As the health hazard of inhaling fibres from the manufacture, use, fabrication and removal of this material has been clearly demonstrated, and because legislation in Great Britain requires the monitoring and control of airborne fibres, it is necessary to establish the airborne concentrations. The procedure for sampling given below is only a summary of a detailed method given in the Health and Safety Executive (HSE) Guidance Note MDHS 39/3, which should be followed closely.

Equipment required for sampling

For each place to be sampled simultaneously: for personal sampling, a sampling pump capable of a flow rate of between 1 and 4 l min^{-1}; for static sampling in asbestos clearance work, a pump capable of up to 8 l min^{-1}; a 25 mm diameter cellulose acetate membrane filter preferably with a gridded surface to assist in focusing on the correct plane for counting; an ERM asbestos type filter holder as shown in Fig. 1.4; one metre of 7 mm internal diameter plastic tubing; a harness for personal sampling or a tripod for static sampling; Petri-slide and forceps or, if the filters are loaded into the holders prior to leaving base, a cover for the filter holder.

Equipment required for counting

Microscope slides and cover glasses; a binocular microscope having phase contrast Koehler illumination and an eyepiece of magnification × 12.5, one eyepiece to contain a Beckett and Walton graticule as illustrated in Fig. 1.21; an HSE/NPL (National Physical Laboratory) phase contrast test slide, an acetone vaporiser, see Fig. 1.20; glycerol triacetate (triacetin); counting forms or two push-button digital counters.

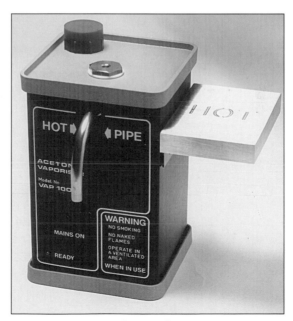

Fig. 1.20. Acetone vaporiser (Casella Ltd).

Method for sampling

The procedure for sampling is the same as for total/inspirable dust as outlined on pages 17–22 except that it is unnecessary to weigh the membrane filter before or after use. The flow rate of the pump will depend upon the volume of air to be sampled. This is set out in detail in HSE Guidance Note EH/10 (rev.) 1995, or more recent notes as they are published (see Table 1.4). The essential features of this guidance are based upon two criteria:

1   For precision the fibre density on the filter should lie on the range 100–400 fibres mm^{-2}.

2   The sample should be representative of the period of exposure being studied.

Method of evaluation

1   Carefully remove membrane filter from the holder or Petri-slide using forceps and place centrally with the gridded side uppermost on a suitably labelled clean microscope slide. Try to have the grids parallel to the side of the slide.

2   Place the slide into the vaporiser according to the manufacturer's instructions and inject the appropriate amount of acetone as advised. The white membrane should now be seen to become transparent as the structure of the membrane collapses under the action of the vapour.

3   Wait for a few minutes to elapse before adding a few drops of triacetin on the cleared membrane and cover with a 25 mm diameter cover glass.

4   The slide should be left for about 24 hours before counting but if a result is required quickly it can be heated to 50 °C for about 15 minutes.

Note: other methods of membrane clearance are available and are detailed in MDHS 39/3.

To estimate the number of respirable fibres on the membrane, proceed as follows:

1   Set up phase contrast lighting conditions on the microscope according to the manufacturer's instructions and check the dimensions of the eyepiece graticule at magnification × 500 by means of a stage micrometer. If the microscope is regularly used for counting then the size of the graticule will be known.

2   Place the slide on the stage of the microscope and focus at a low magnification to observe the distribution of fibres over the whole slide and to determine whether the fibres are evenly distributed or not.

3   Change to × 500 magnification and check the performance of the microscope using the HSE/NPL phase contrast test slide Mk 2 making sure that block 5 on the slide can be seen. Adjust the

Table 1.4. Examples of approximate sample densities produced by various concentrations, flow rates and sampling times

Possible application	Concentration (fibres ml^{-1})	Flow rates (l min^{-1})	Sampling time	Sample volume (l)	Sample density (fibres mm^{-2})
Clearance indicator	0.01	8	60 (min)	480	12.6
Clearance indicator	0.01	8	4 (h)	1920	50
Action level	0.1	2	4 (h)	480	126
Action level	0.25	2	4 (h)	480	315
4 h control limit	0.2	1	4 (h)	240	126
4 h control limit	0.5	1	4 (h)	240	315
10 min control limit	0.6	4	10 (min)	40	63
10 min control limit	1.5	4	10 (min)	40	158

From HSE Guidance Note EH/10.

microscope according to the manufacturer's instructions to achieve this.

4 Remove the test slide and place the slide to be counted on the stage. Select a field of view at random and count the number of respirable fibres present in the circle of the graticule. It may be necessary to slightly alter the position of the focus up and down in order to ensure that any fibres out of focus can be seen. Rules for counting fibres that lay across the boundaries of the graticule, for split fibres and fibre bundles, are detailed in HSE MDHS 39/3, which should always be consulted before sampling and counting.

Note: a respirable fibre is defined as: one that is greater than 5 μm in length and having a length/breadth ratio of at least 3:1 and a diameter less than 3 μm. The blocks and lines around the outside of the Beckett and Walton graticule in Fig. 1.21 assist in selecting the correct fibres to count.

5 Having decided upon the number of fibres present in the field, note it on the counting form or the digital counter, randomly change the field of view, and repeat. Normally 100 fields of view should be counted unless 200 fibres have been seen in fewer than that. However, at least 20 fields must be counted whatever the number seen.

Note: if the distribution of fibres on the membrane is seen to be uneven or if the number of fibres present is low the fields of view should be chosen in a viewing pattern as shown in Fig. 1.22.

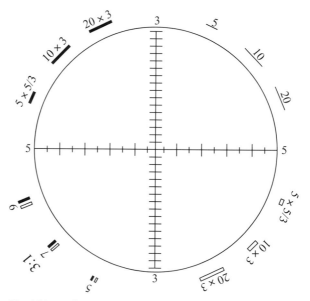

Fig. 1.21. Beckett and Walton graticule.

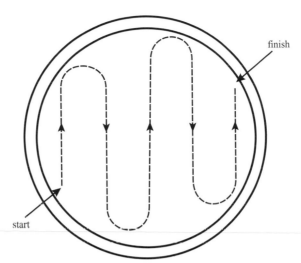

Fig. 1.22. A viewing pattern for scanning asbestos slides to ensure the whole filter is viewed to obtain a true average.

Calculations

Let:

D (mm) = effective diameter of the membrane (i.e. the actual diameter less the overlap due to the retaining ring of the filter holder)

d (mm) = the diameter of each field of view

n = the number of fields examined

N = the number of fibres counted

V (ml) = the volume of air sampled.

V = flow rate of pump ($1 \min^{-1}$) × duration of sampling (min) × 1000 ml.

$$\text{Estimated number of fibres sampled} = \frac{D^2}{d^2} \times \frac{N}{n} \text{ fibres}$$

$$\text{Fibre concentration} = \frac{\text{estimated number of fibres}}{V} \text{ fibres ml}^{-1}$$

The results obtained should be compared with the *Control Limits* published in EH/10. Paragraphs 8 and 9 are reproduced below:

> 8 The Control Limits to be used depend upon the type of asbestos which is present. The limits are more stringent if amosite or crocidolite (or both) are present than if they are not. For each of the two categories there are two limits: one is a limit on the average dust level over any continuous 4 hour period, and the other is a limit on the average level over any continuous 10 minute period. Each is a Control Limit in its own right.

9 The *Control Limits* are
    (a)   for asbestos consisting of or containing any crocidolite or amosite:
        (i)   0.2 fibres per millilitre of air averaged over any continuous period of 4 hours;
        (ii)   0.6 fibres per millilitre of air averaged over any continuous period of 10 minutes;
    (b)   for asbestos consisting of or containing other types of asbestos but not crocidolite or amosite:
        (i)   0.5 fibres per millilitre of air averaged over any continuous period of 4 hours;
        (ii)   1.5 fibres per millilitre of air averaged over any continuous period of 10 minutes.
Employers may choose to assume that the asbestos is amosite or crocidolite and that the more stringent limits apply; identification of the type of asbestos is then unnecessary.

Possible problems
1   The field may be heavily contaminated with other dust, thus making it difficult to see the fibres. In this case reduce the sampling flow rate or reduce the sampling time.
2   To ensure that the plane of view is correctly focussed, always use a membrane which has a gridded surface and focus on the grid lines.
3   Accuracy in counting is increased by spending as long as possible on each field.
4   Care must be taken to ensure absolute cleanliness throughout to prevent unwanted contamination of the sample.
5   Inter-person/laboratory counting should normally be employed to indicate individual variations in counting characteristics.
For man-made mineral fibres (MMMF) please see MDHS59.

The choice of filter and filter holder to suit a specific dust, fume or mist
When sampling for a specific dust of known composition or type it is important to consult the analyst before starting as the method of analysis will vary for the different chemical composition of the dust. Each method will require the dust to be presented in a partic-ular way and the analyst will advise as to the best filter to use to suit the technique being applied. Table 1.5 gives some of the more commonly encountered dusts and the recommended filter to use.
    When a cyclone is used to separate the respirable or alveolar dust it is important to ensure that the correct air-flow rate is passing to suit the type of selector being used and that the flow rate is not pulsating.

Table 1.5. Details of filters and filter holders to be used for various types of dust

Type of dust	Method of analysis	Filter required*	Filter holder required
Asbestos fibres	Optical microscopy	Cellulose ester*	ERM type (Fig. 1.3)
	Scanning electron microscopy	Nuclepore	ERM type (Fig. 1.3)
	X-ray diffraction	Silver membrane	ERM type (Fig. 1.3)
Man-made fibres	Optical microscopy	Cellulose ester*	ERM type (Fig. 1.3)
	Gravimetric	Glass fibre	(Fig. 1.2a, b or c)
Silica	X-ray diffraction	Silver membrane or glass fibre	Cyclone (Fig. 1.5, 1.18 ir 1.19)
	Infrared	Polyvinyl chloride	Cyclone (Fig. 1.5, 1.18 ir 1.19)
Lead, heavy metals, their oxides and salts	Atomic adsorption spectroscopy	Cellulose ester or glass fibre	(Fig. 1.4)
Nuisance and general	Gravimetric	Glass fibre	(Fig. 1.2a, b or c)
	Optical microscopy	Cellulose ester	(Fig. 1.2a, b or c)
Unknown dusts	X-ray diffraction	Silver membrane	(Fig. 1.2a, b or c)
Coal	Gravimetric	Glass fibre	Cyclone or MRE 113 (Fig. 1.2 or 1.6)
Coal with rock	Infrared	Polyvinyl chloride	Cyclone or MRE 113 (Fig. 1.2 or 1.6)
	X-ray diffraction	Silver membrane	Cyclone or MRE 113 (Fig. 1.2 or 1.6)
Oil mists	Gravimetric	Glass fibre	Open face
	Fluorescent spectroscopy	Cellulose ester*	Open face
Welding fume	Gravimetric	Cellulose ester*	(Fig. 1.2a, b or c)
	Atomic adsorption spectroscopy	Cellulose ester*	(Fig. 1.2a, b or c)

* Note that where cellulose ester membranes are used the pore size should be 0.8 µm.
ERM = European Reference Method.

To take a sample, proceed as with the total/inhalable dust or the cyclone separator methods described previously but using the type of filter and holder detailed in Table 1.5.

To trace the behaviour of a dust cloud using a Tyndall beam

Aim

Many particles of dust are too small to see with the naked eye under normal lighting conditions but when a beam of strong light is passed through a cloud of particles they reflect the light to the observer and as a result become readily visible. A natural occurrence of this phenomenon is observed when a shaft of sunlight shines into a dark building highlighting the airborne particles. The scientist J. Tyndall made use of this principle to observe the behaviour of dust clouds using a beam of light and his name has been associated with the technique from that time on. Thus, if a portable lamp having a strong parallel beam is set up to shine through an environment suspected of being dusty the movement of the particles can be observed. Although no numerical measurements are normally made, the performance of extract ventilation systems associated with dust-emitting processes can be watched and design corrections made if unsatisfactory capture is noticed. It may be useful to film or video record the occurrence.

Equipment required

A strong mains- or battery-powered parallel-beamed lamp (a car spotlight is suitable; a foglight is not), a tripod stand for mounting the lamp and a black screen. There is a Tyndall beam apparatus commercially available in a portable kit form which has a lamp reflector designed to provide a strong parallel beam of light (Fig. 1.23).

Method

Set up the lamp and screen as shown in Fig. 1.24 with the observer in the position indicated. When the lamp is switched on the dust cloud should be clearly seen and the movement of the particles observed, photographed or filmed. The best position of the lamp and screen may have to be adjusted by trial and error but it is important to shield the lamp from the eyes of the observer or the camera to prevent glare.

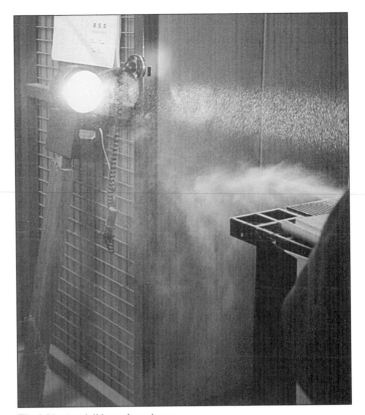

Fig. 1.23. Tyndall beam lamp in use.

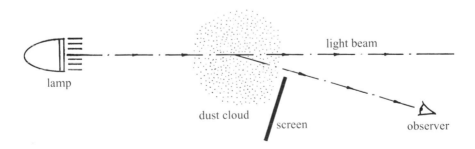

Fig. 1.24. Layout of Tyndall beam apparatus in relation to a dust cloud (A & G Marketing).

Further reading

American Conference of Government Industrial Hygienists (1977) *Air Sampling Instruments Manual*. ACGIH, Cincinnati.

Health and Safety Executive (1986) *Control of Lead: Air Sampling Techniques and Strategies*. Guidance Note EH28. HSE Books, Sudbury, Suffolk.

Health and Safety Executive (1989) *Man-made Mineral Fibres in Air*. Guidance Note MDHS 59. HMSO, London.

Health and Safety Executive (1995) *Asbestos: Exposure Limits and Measurement of Airborne Dust Concentrations*. Guidance Note EH10 (Rev.). HSE Books, Sudbury, Suffolk.

Health and Safety Executive (1996) *Asbestos Fibres in Air. Light Microscope Methods for Use with the Control of Asbestos at Work Regulations 1995*. Guidance Note MDHS39/4 (Rev.). HSE Books, Sudbury, Suffolk.

Health and Safety Executive (1997) *General methods for sampling and gravimetric analysis of respirable and total inhalable dust*. Guidance Note MDHS 14/2, HSE Books, Sudbury, Suffolk.

Health and Safety Executive (1997) *The Dust Lamp: a Simple Tool for Observing the Presence of Airborne Particles*. Guidance Note MDHS82. HSE Books, Sudbury, Suffolk.

Lee, G.L. (1980) Sampling: principles, apparatus, surveys. In: *Occupational Hygiene* (eds H.A. Waldron & J.M. Harrington), pp. 39–60. Blackwell Scientific Publications, Oxford.

Mark, D. (1995) The sampling of aerosols: principles and methods. In: *Occupational Hygiene* (eds J.M. Harrington & K. Gardiner), pp. 99–122. Blackwell Science, Oxford.

SI 1999 No. 437 and Approved Code of Practice (1999) *Control of Substances Hazardous to Health Regulations*. HMSO, London.

Vincent, I. & Brosseau, L.M. (1995) The nature and properties of workplace airborne contaminants. In: *Occupational Hygiene* (eds J.M. Harrington & K. Gardiner), pp. 61–83. Blackwell Science, Oxford.

Walton W.H. & Beckett S.T. (1977) A microscope eyepiece graticule for the evaluation of fibrous dusts. *Annals of Occupational Hygiene* **20**, 19–23.

2 Gases and vapours

Introduction

Many industrial processes as well as natural or biological degradation processes utilise or produce gas, often under pressure. Containing these gases is a major problem since many are toxic or may cause asphyxia in enclosed environments. Leaks may occur around joints, valves, or through piping, and access covers when opened release gas into the atmosphere. Therefore, suitable precautions have to be taken to contain these gases and their presence in the atmosphere around these containers has to be monitored.

Solvents are another source of respirable materials. These are liquids chosen for their ability to dissolve a particular material and often for their ability to evaporate and dissociate themselves from the solute. In so doing, a vapour is formed and it is unfortunate that the majority of solvents have biological activities. Most have a narcotic effect acting upon the central nervous system slowing down nerve responses; others are extremely toxic or are sensitising agents; and some can be mutagenic and/or carcinogenic.

The range of gases and vapours that occur in industry, commerce, medicine, agriculture and in the home and street is vast, requiring a wide variety of monitoring and detection techniques. A few methods of sampling and detection are described in this chapter. The techniques available fall into two basic types: (1) direct measurement of concentrations or indication of presence with instruments or detection devices; and (2) indirect analysis of pollutant or air collected from the workplace and examined in a laboratory. The satisfactory use of many of the instruments available requires a good knowledge of chemistry and is best left to those trained in analytical chemistry, but colorimetric detector tubes and paper tape monitors can be used by any competent individual. Certain collection devices can also be straightforward to use provided the analysis is left to someone experienced.

As with airborne dust measurement, if a time-weighted average concentration is required then it is usual to collect a sample of the gas/vapour laden air over the working period rather than use a direct reading instrument, which usually takes an instantaneous measurement or 'grab sample'. Some direct reading instruments, however, do have recorders attached to them so that peaks and troughs of concentration can be seen and averages calculated. Some are linked to data loggers or computers so that printout facilities can provide information in accordance with a pre-programmed format. These devices produce general workroom levels of concentration as it is

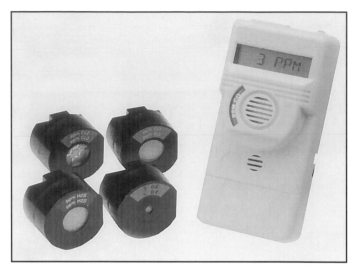

Fig. 2.1. Personal gas detector (Casella Ltd).

difficult to attach them to employees to estimate their personal exposure from the breathing zone. However, for a limited number of gases, specially designed long-term detector tubes that can be used as personal samplers are now available. Furthermore, there are personal gas detectors on the market that use interchangeable precalibrated sensor blocks capable of singly detecting many gases, mainly inorganic. They produce a real-time direct reading display loading down to a 48-hour on-board data logger. One such device is illustrated in Fig. 2.1.

As mentioned above, sampling for airborne chemicals can be done in two ways: by collecting continuously a small amount of the workroom atmosphere, gradually filling a container over the test period; or by allowing workroom air to pass through an adsorbent material such as activated charcoal. This will adsorb certain gases, which can later be desorbed in a more concentrated form for analysis. In the first case the receptacle will contain a sample of the workroom atmosphere, which represents the average mixture of all gases present at the sampling position over the period sampled. Unless the sampling air-flow rate is low the final sample can be quite bulky. With the adsorbent method of collection the pollutant is concentrated, which makes analysis more reliable.

Equipment available

Collection devices
Before embarking upon any form of air sampling it is important to discuss with the analyst which method of collection best suits the analytical technique to be employed when the samples are returned

to the laboratory. The method of analysis dictates the type of container or collection device to be used, as the final sample has to be introduced into the analytical instrument.

Containers

If a sample of the workroom air is required for complete analysis – that is, for the normal constituents of fresh air, oxygen, nitrogen and carbon dioxide; and for certain pollutants such as carbon monoxide, sulphur dioxide, oxides of nitrogen and some hydrocarbons such as methane – then it can be collected in a container to be returned to the laboratory. But if other gases and vapours need to be known and are sampled in a container there is a risk that some pollutants may be adsorbed on the walls of the container and not released when required for analysis, and some may well be released at a later time when the container is being used again. Therefore, there are some risks with this method, and some knowledge of the behaviour of the gases to be sampled and the materials of construction of the container is required.

Samples can be collected in: metal cylinders, syringes, glass or plastic pipettes and plastic or rubber bags. For grab samples they can be filled by hand pump. For long-term samples bags should be used as they can be filled slowly over the sampling period by a small battery-powered pump.

One disadvantage with the container method of sampling is that it is difficult to obtain a personal sample as most receptacles are rather bulky or are only suited to grab sampling. Another disadvantage is that the sample collected contains the pollutant at the average concentration at which it occurs at the sampling point. This may be very low, thus the analytical equipment used to determine the concentration must be very sensitive.

Adsorption methods

Certain gases and vapours are readily adsorbed by solid materials such as silica gel, activated charcoal and various types of porous resin. When air containing those gases or vapours is passed through the material they will be adsorbed. Tubes of metal or glass can be made or purchased containing one of these materials. The tubes should remain sealed until ready for use.* When a continuous stream of air is passed through them by means of an air pump the material will adsorb those gases or vapours for which they are designed. Provided that the amount of air passed through has not over-loaded the adsorbent then the amount of pollutant collected can be determined in the laboratory and an average concentration

---

* Adsorbent tubes must not be confused with colorimetric detector tubes.

calculated knowing the amount of air passed through the monitoring device.

One advantage of this technique is that the pumps and tubes are small and can be attached to an employee in a similar way to the airborne dust samplers. Another advantage is that the pollutant is collected in a concentrated form, thus analytical techniques need be less sensitive than with the container methods, and several gases or vapours can be collected and analysed from the same tube.

Not all gases or vapours can be collected by means of the adsorbent tube. Another technique available is to bubble the workroom air through water or some liquid in which the gas is soluble. The analyst then deals with the gas in solution. The container for the liquid is known as an impinger or 'bubbler' because the sampled air is introduced via a tube whose end is below the surface of the liquid; thus the air is bubbled through it. Unfortunately most bubblers need to be kept upright to prevent the reagent from spilling out. This limits their use for personal sampling because employees wearing them are not able to bend or stoop. Another disadvantage of this technique is that it is difficult to guarantee that all the gas passing through the bubbler will be absorbed, as bubbling does not ensure 100 per cent contact between the gas and the liquid. To improve contact 'fritted bubblers' are used, which have an inlet tube whose end is of porous glass producing very small bubbles.

Passive samplers

Techniques are available whereby adsorbent material can be used to sample concentrations of airborne pollutants without using a pump to draw air through the collector. The adsorbent material, which can be liquid or solid, is contained in a holder designed to allow the gases to diffuse and/or permeate to the adsorbent surface. These holders are small enough to be worn like a lapel badge (Fig. 2.2) or tube (Fig. 2.3) and are free of any pump or tubing. At the end of the sampling period the holder is returned to the laboratory where the amount of gas or vapour collected can be analysed as with adsorbent tubes.

The advantages of this type of sampling are as follows:

1   It removes the need for a costly pump, with the associated problems of flow rates, battery state and worker resistance to use.
2   The samplers are light and unobtrusive.
3   There is a constant sampling rate.

Pumps

When slowly filling bags, and for drawing air through adsorbent tubes, a low air-flow rate is required. Pumps are available that provide rates as low as 2 millilitres per minute (ml min^{-1}) but the range for this type of sampling is between 2 and 500 ml min^{-1}.

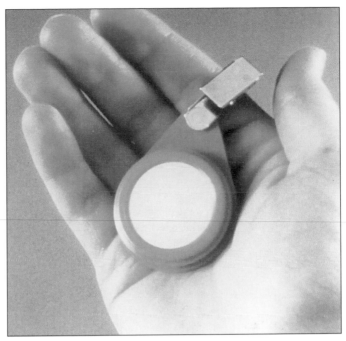

Fig. 2.2. Passive sampler (3M UK Ltd).

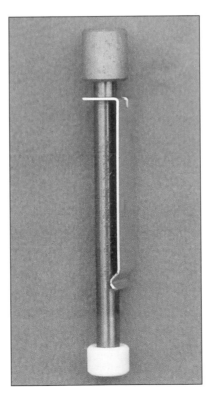

Fig. 2.3. Diffusive sampler
(Casella Ltd).

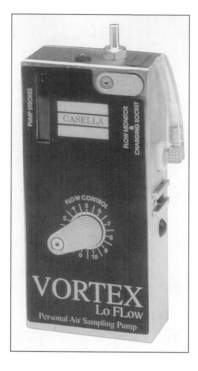

Fig. 2.4. Low flow-rate sampling pump (Casella Ltd).

These pumps operate under the same principles as the dust sampling pumps, that is, diaphragm, piston and rotary, and, with certain exceptions, are supplied by the same manufacturers (Fig. 2.4). The correct flow rate to use is influenced by the airborne concentration of the pollutant, the ability of the material to adsorb, the size of the sampling tube and the duration of sampling. Bubblers tend to require higher flow rates therefore the medium-flow pumps as used in dust sampling are preferred.

Most pumps available have a variable flow control either by means of varying the stroke of the diaphragm or by varying the speed of the driving motor. One pump, however, operates by providing a suction through a 'critical orifice', which limits the amount of air flowing through it, a change in flow rate being achieved by changing the size of the orifice. Flow rates of any pump should always be checked against a soap bubble flowmeter or a calibrated rotameter (see Chapter 1).

Tube holders

In order to hold the adsorbent tube and to attach it to an employee if required, a tube holder is available from the suppliers of the low flow-rate pumps. A piece of flexible plastic tubing connects the holder to the pump.

Adsorbent tubes

The materials that are used for adsorbing gases and vapours are listed as follows: charcoal, silica gel, alumina, various porous polymers under the names of; Poropak P, Poropak Q, Chromosorb 101, Chromosorb 102 and Tenax GC. They each have the ability to adsorb various gases and vapours but charcoal is the most widely used as it has an adsorbent affinity with more substances than any other material. The materials are contained in either glass or metal tubes depending upon the method of desorbing the gas in the laboratory. One method involves breaking the tube so that the adsorbent material falls into a liquid that leaches the gas out of the material into solution. Glass tubes are used in this application. Another method involves heating the tube to drive off the collected gas into a detection system. Metal tubes are used for this technique. Tubes can be made up in the laboratory or purchased.

The tubes designed for solvent leaching are made up in two sections to indicate what is known as 'breakthrough'. This occurs when the sorbent material is completely saturated with the sampled gases. If the second section of the tube is free of the sampled gases then breakthrough has not occurred in the first section and the total sample collected on that section can be used in the calculation for airborne concentration. Breakthrough occurs when the sample volume is too high or the sample duration is too long to suit the airborne concentration in the sampling position.

With metal tubes for thermal desorption no second section can be applied, thus breakthrough must be carefully guarded against by calculation of breakthrough volumes not to be exceeded during sampling. For more details see Thain (1980).

It cannot be emphasised too strongly that, when sampling for airborne gases and vapours, the analyst who undertakes the analysis of the collected samples must advise on the best sampling method. If adsorbent tubes are to be used, he/she will advise on the sorbent material and sample volumes that should be used.

Colorimetric detector tubes

A comparatively simple method to detect airborne gases uses the detector tube. This consists of a glass tube containing crystals treated with a chemical reagent which will react with a particular gas and change colour as a result. As contaminated air is drawn through the tube a colour change occurs from the inlet end which extends along the tube, depending upon the concentration of the gas present. A scale is printed on the side of the tube and the measured concentration is indicated by the length of stain for a particular sample volume. A hand-operated suction pump or calibrated syringe ensures the appropriate sample volume passes through if operated according to the maker's instructions. The tubes are sealed

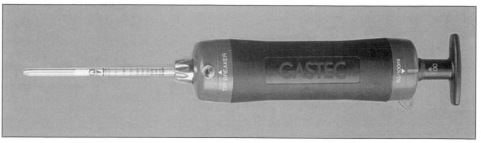

Fig. 2.5. Colorimetric detector tube pump (Anachem Ltd).

at each end and both ends must be broken before inserting into the pump. An example of this type of sampler is shown in Fig. 2.5. Two companies specialise in these devices – Dräger and Gastec – and between them detector tubes for over 200 substances are available. The tubes supplied by these companies are not interchangeable, that is, Gastec tubes cannot be used with a Dräger pump and vice versa.

Whilst the technique appears simple there are certain difficulties that can lead to error in the results obtained. The detector tubes deteriorate with time and have a shelf life of no more than 2 years if stored at normal room temperatures. The presence of other gases can interfere with the gas to be measured. The manufacturer will advise in these cases. Also, it is important that the designed sample volume passes through the tube otherwise the result will be invalid. This means that any damage to the pump or syringe causing a leak in the air flow will reduce the volume of air passing through the tube.

It is possible to obtain a time-weighted average concentration by means of a colorimetric detector tube for certain gases listed later in this chapter. The technique involves using a battery-powered sampling pump and drawing air through the tube, which is placed in the breathing zone of the worker. It should be noted that sampling must be undertaken with purpose-made long-running tubes, i.e. short-term tubes cannot be used for this type of sampling.

Direct reading instruments

There are many direct reading instruments on the market that are specific to a particular gas such as carbon monoxide, sulphur dioxide or mercury vapour. Most of them can be coupled to a chart recorder to obtain a continuous record of the peaks and troughs of exposure concentrations, which can be very useful for relating the job being undertaken with the concentration at any moment. Unfortunately, they are normally quite bulky and unsuitable for personal sampling unless an inlet tube can be attached to the worker to draw air from the breathing zone and the instrument carried close to the worker. If several gases require to be measured by direct means it can become quite expensive to buy an instrument for each one. However, there are several types of instrument available, which can be used to measure a range of gases and vapours. One of these, the Organic Vapour Analyser (OVA), is a portable battery-powered gas chromatograph with a flame ionisation detector (Fig. 2.6). This will either indicate total hydrocarbon concentration or, if fitted with a suitable column, will indicate the concentrations of specific vapours.

Another, the Miran infrared analyser, is capable of emitting infrared light in a range of wavelengths into a detection chamber through which the sampled gas can be continuously drawn by means of an integral pump (Fig. 2.7). Infrared light of the detection wavelength is absorbed by the gas or vapour present in proportion to the concentration present and this is indicated on a meter, or the signal can be fed into a data-logger or continuous chart recorder.

A third type of instrument uses paper tape impregnated with a chemical that changes colour when in contact with a specific gas producing, on the paper, a stain whose intensity varies with the

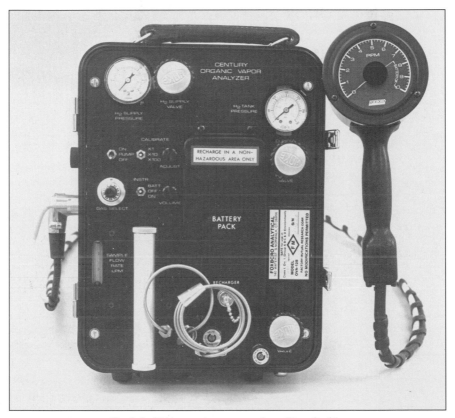

Fig. 2.6. OVA organic vapour analyser (Quantitech).

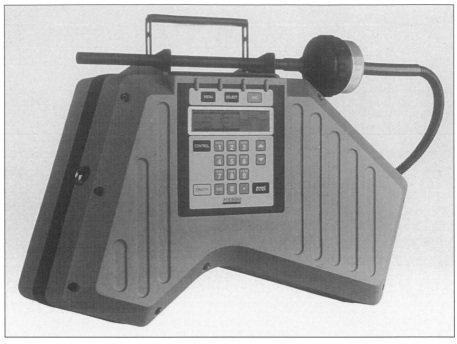

Fig. 2.7. MIRAN SapphIRe Portable infrared gas analyser (Quantitech).

concentration of the gas present. This is then indicated by shining a beam of light through it. The intensity of the beam is diminished by the stain and detected by a photomultiplier. The paper tapes are held in a 'chemcassette', which can be changed when full or when a different gas is to be detected. Such an instrument by MDA Scientific is shown in Fig. 2.8.

General

The range of instruments available is so large that it is impossible to cover them in a book of this nature. The instruments specific to particular gases and the paper-tape types are generally easy to use and good instructions are always provided by the manufacturers. The tunable infrared instruments and the portable chromatograph types require a good knowledge of chemistry to obtain reliable results.

To obtain a personal sample for solvent vapours using an adsorbent tube

Aim

In order to obtain a time-weighted average concentration of the exposure of an employee to solvent vapours it is necessary to collect

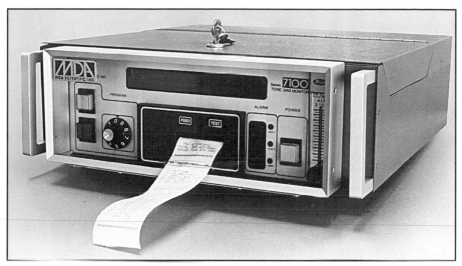

Fig. 2.8. Paper tape sampler (MDA).

a representative sample of the air from his or her breathing zone over the period of exposure. This can be achieved by adsorbing the vapour on to a medium such as charcoal. Other media are available but the analytical chemist will advise as to the most suitable for the vapours in question.

Equipment required
A low flow-rate pump; an adsorbent tube; a tube holder with a length of plastic tubing to connect to the pump; a calibrated rotameter or portable soap bubble calibrator (Fig. 2.9); and a harness may also be useful.

Method
1   Break the glass seals or remove the covers at each end of the tube packed with adsorbent and insert into the holder. Connect the other end of the tube to the pump.
2   Attach the tube holder to the worker as close to the breathing zone as possible, the lapel or clothing close to the collar bone being the most acceptable place. Place the pump in a convenient pocket or hang from the worker's belt.
3   Turn on the pump and note the time of starting.
4   Some pumps are fitted with a stroke counter and the reading on the counter must be noted before starting. Also, these are fitted with an orifice to provide the correct flow rate. Check that this orifice is the one recommended by the manufacturer for the flow rate required. With other types of pump check the flow rate with a calibrated flowmeter or rotameter and note its value. Advice

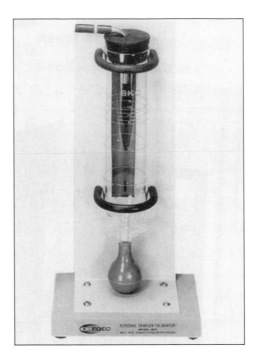

Fig. 2.9. Portable soap bubble calibrator (SKC Ltd).

should have been obtained from an analyst, or a calculation should have been carried out to determine the appropriate flow rate, after taking into account the concentration of vapours expected and the length of the sampling period.

5 From time to time during the operation check the flow rate for constancy using the rotameter or a soap bubble flowmeter.

6 At the end of the period stop the pump and note the time and the reading on the stroke counter where applicable.

7 Remove the apparatus from the worker and place seals at the open ends of the adsorbent tube. Label the tube for identification purposes.

8 Send the tube to the analyst with information concerning the substances likely to be adsorbed on the medium and which require analysis.

Calculations

It is first necessary to establish how much air has passed through the tube. The calculation to do this will depend on the type of pump used. With pumps having a stroke counter ascertain the total number of strokes that occurred during the sampling period by subtracting the first reading from the second and multiplying the result by the displacement value of each stroke as advised by the manufacturer for the setting or orifice used. Convert the results to cubic metres, that is, if the result is in ml min^{-1} multiply that value by the total number of minutes that elapsed during the sampling period and divide by 10^6.

After the adsorbent tube has been analysed the total amount of each vapour tested will be given in milligrams (mg) or micrograms (μg). Divide the weight given by the total sampled volume to give the concentration in mg m^{-3} or μg m^{-3}.

Example

A pump passing 5 ml min^{-1} sampled an atmosphere for 6 hours 40 minutes using a charcoal adsorbing tube in a workplace polluted with paint solvents. The analyst reported that the sample contained the following amounts of solvent: 1-butanol, 0.156 mg; xylene, 0.298 mg; styrene, 0.187 mg. Calculate the airborne concentrations of each.

Total time of sampling = $6 \times 60 + 40 = 400$ min.

Total airflow through tube at 5 ml min^{-1} = $5 \times 400 = 2000$ ml = 0.002 m^3 *

Concentrations:

$$1\text{-Butanol} = \frac{0.156}{0.002} = 78\,\text{mg m}^{-3}$$

$$\text{Xylene} = \frac{0.298}{0.002} = 149\,\text{mg m}^{-3}$$

$$\text{Styrene} = \frac{0.187}{0.002} = 93.5\,\text{mg m}^{-3}$$

Possible problems

The problem of 'breakthrough' must be guarded against. This occurs when the adsorbent material has been overloaded. After sampling for a period of time the adsorbent can become saturated with the vapour and no more can be collected, thus making continued sampling pointless. It is not always possible to know when this happens. It may occur when the sampling rate is too high or the concentration of vapours upon which the rate has been based has been under-estimated. Some proprietary tubes contain a second stage that is analysed separately from the first. If this second stage contains no adsorbed vapour then breakthrough has not occurred and the first stage holds all the sample. If there is some doubt about the range of concentration that is likely to occur in the workplace,

---

* It must be pointed out that the most inaccurate part of this or any similar test lies with the flow rate of the pump, which could be as much as ± 10% in error. Therefore, it is unwise to be pedantic about the decimal point in the result.

therefore giving rise to uncertainty as to whether breakthrough could occur, then a second adsorbent tube should be added to the first in series by means of a short piece of plastic tubing. Each tube should then be analysed separately. A further precaution can be employed by adding two 'two-stage' tubes in series thus providing four stages of adsorption. Provided that the last stage is free of vapour when analysed then it can be confidently assumed that all the vapour has been collected in the previous stages. The total vapour collection on all stages must be used in the calculation. To avoid breakthrough, provided a reasonable estimate of the airborne concentration of the vapours is known, the analyst can advise on the flow rates and sampling duration. Alternatively these can be calculated knowing the degree of precision of the analytical equipment.

The collection of gases using a sampling bag

Aim
It is possible to obtain a time-weighted average concentration of an airborne gas by passing it through a detector of a direct reading instrument from a bag, which can be filled over a timed period. The resulting mixture in the bag will be a mean of the peaks and troughs of the concentrations occurring during the period. Therefore, if some of the collected sample is introduced into the direct reading instrument the time-weighted average concentration will be indicated. Due to the bulk of the bag it is difficult, but not impossible, to obtain a personal sample.

Equipment required
A low flow-rate sampling pump, a bag (see Fig. 2.10) and a length of connecting tubing. As most sampling pumps are designed for suction only a few are fitted with a discharge nozzle to which tubing can be attached. For this operation it is essential to choose a pump with that facility. With the Casella Lo Flow pump it is possible to fit a nozzle to the discharge port.

The flow rate should be as low as possible in order to make the sampling period as long as possible and to keep the size of the bag to manageable proportions. If the pump is capable of a flow rate of, say, 5 ml min^{-1} then during the course of eight hours it will have passed some 2400 ml of sample or 2.4 l, which represents a bag of approximately 13.5 cm^3. However, if the pump handles 500 ml min^{-1} for 8 hours the sample would amount to 240 l, requiring a bag of 62 cm^3, which would be much more difficult to manage. Table 2.1 gives the total volume collected for various periods and for various flow rates.

The bags should be of strong non-porous plastic with welded seams and a single supply tube with some means of closing it.

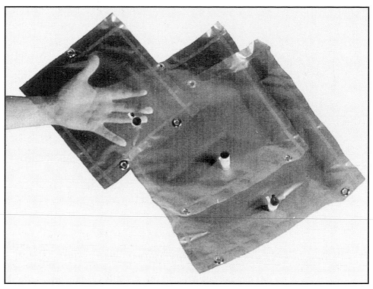

Fig. 2.10. Sampling bags (SKC Ltd)

Specially designed sampling bags are available made of a variety of plastics some having aluminium impregnated into the pores to minimise leakage and surface retention.

Table 2.1. Total collected volume of sample for various flow rates and sampling duration

Flow rate (ml min^{-1})	Total sampled volume in litres				Remarks on manageability
	1 hour	2 hour	4 hour	8 hour	
2	0.12	0.24	0.48	0.96	Could be worn by an employee
5	0.30	0.60	1.20	2.40	
10	0.60	1.20	2.40	4.80	Too large to be worn by an employee but one person could transport four
50	3.00	6.00	12.00	24.00	
100	6.00	12.00	24.00	48.00	Much too large to be worn and only one could be reasonably transported by one person
200	12.00	24.00	48.00	96.00	
500	30.00	60.00	120.00	240.00	
1000	60.00	120.00	240.00	480.00	

Method
1 Completely deflate the bag having ensured that it has been flushed through at least four times with clean air to remove or dilute any previous sample.

2   If no valve is fitted to the supply tube then fit a tube clamp to it.

3   Connect the bag to the discharge nozzle of the pump via suitably sized tubing.

4   Set up the assembly at the point of sampling, either on an employee if a very low flow-rate pump is being used or in a static position. For static sampling it is useful to attach the pump and tubing to a tripod by means of adhesive tape or string. For personal sampling a bag holder and harness are available.

5   Open the bag valve or unclamp the supply tube and start the pump, noting the time.

6   Adjust the flow rate of the pump to suit the size of the bag and the sampling period, i.e. larger bags can take higher flow rates. It is not important to know the exact flow rate.

7   Stop the pump after the sampling period is completed and seal the valve or clamp the tube, noting the time.

8   Immediately transport the bag to the direct reading instrument, which should have been warmed up if necessary, zeroed and calibrated in readiness. The instrument preparations should be done strictly in accordance with the manufacturer's instructions. It is important to analyse the sample as quickly as possible as even the best sampling bags are slightly porous and the sample can diffuse away or change its composition.

Results

The reading obtained on the instrument is the time-weighted average concentration of the pollutant measured.

Sampling for gases using a bubbler

Aim

Some gases are not readily adsorbed by solids but dissolve in liquids or form chemical reactions with certain reagents when in contact. One method of introduction is to bubble the workroom air through the appropriate liquid using a device called a bubbler or impinger. Time-weighted average concentrations can be obtained by allowing the bubbling action to continue for a period of time. The success of this technique depends upon the readiness of the pollutant in question to react with the solution or reagent. Unfortunately the nature of bubbles is such that not all the gas may come into contact with the liquid, thus some of the pollutant can escape. To overcome this, some bubblers are designed to produce very fine bubbles using a device known as a frit. Also, bubblers can be staged in series so that as the air leaves the first it then passes into a second or even a third stage.

Clearly, devices such as these are unwieldy to use particularly if a personal sample is to be obtained from the breathing zone of an employee and there is a risk that the liquid may be spilt if not kept upright. A spill-proof bubbler is available; nevertheless, obvious resistance from the workforce to wearing devices containing what may be dangerous chemicals is likely to be encountered. Bubbling techniques are therefore usually confined to static workplace sampling rather than personal.

Equipment required

A bubbler containing the correct amount of appropriate liquid as advised by the analytical chemist, a suction pump, connecting tubing, a tripod stand, adhesive tape, a calibrated rotameter, and, if the atmosphere to be sampled is dusty, then an open-face filter holder containing a glass-fibre filter should be added at the entrance to the sampling train.

Method

In order to establish the required pump flow rate it is important to have a trial run beforehand using clean water in the bubbler, the amount being the same as that required for the test. This is to ensure that no liquid is unintentionally drawn into the pump thus causing damage. If the bubbler is filled beforehand and carried to the site it must be kept upright and the open ends sealed. It may be more convenient to fill on site but that involves carrying a measuring device to monitor the correct amount of liquid.

1 Connect the bubbler to the pump, that is, connect the pump to the tube not in contact with the liquid. *Do not connect the pump to the central tube.*

2 At the sampling site attach the assembly to the tripod stand by means of adhesive tape or suitable clamps.

3 Start the pump at the pre-set rate of flow, noting the time.

4 Using a calibrated flowmeter or rotameter check and note the air-flow rate passing through the train and repeat from time to time throughout the test.

5 At the end of the sampling period stop the pump and note the time.

6 Disconnect the tubing from the bubbler, seal its ends and label it.

7 Return the bubbler to the laboratory immediately so that analysis can proceed without delay as some chemicals can change in a short period of time.

Calculation
Establish the total amount of air that has passed through the sampler by multiplying the elapsed time by the flow. Convert to cubic metres (m^3). The analyst will report the amount of pollutant collected in milligrams (mg) or micrograms (μg) and from that the airborne concentration can be obtained in mg m^{-3} or μg m^{-3} by dividing the sample amount by the total flow volume.

Example
A bubbler was run for 20 minutes at a flow rate of 1.5 l min^{-1} in an atmosphere containing formaldehyde. The analyst reported that the sample contained 0.048 mg of formaldehyde. Determine the airborne concentration.

Total airflow through the bubbler $= 20 \times 1.5 = 30$ l $= 0.03$ m^3

$$\text{Airborne concentration of formaldehyde} = \frac{0.048}{0.03} = 1.6 \, \text{mg m}^{-3}$$

To measure the short-term airborne concentration of a gas using a colorimetric detector tube

Aim
It is often necessary to obtain a quick indication of an airborne concentration of a gas. This may be required in a situation such as checking the concentration in an enclosed space, a sump or a large empty vessel before permitting persons to enter. It is also useful in a workplace or workroom to check the general concentration of a specific gas from time to time. Short-term detector tubes can be used for this purpose but it must be remembered that these devices give an indication over a short period of time, usually less than one minute. The exact time taken to produce the result depends upon the type of gas to be detected and type of tube being used and is governed by the flow resistance of the tube. In occupational hygiene parlance this is known as a 'grab' sample and does not provide a time-weighted average concentration. For certain gases a long-term detector tube is available, which is used in a long-term sampling apparatus (see Fig. 2.15) and which should not be confused with a short-term tube.

Equipment required
A colorimetric sampling kit containing a hand-operated suction pump and, from the same manufacturer, a box of detector tubes for the gas to be measured and of the range of concentrations likely to be found. If sumps and enclosed vessels, or difficult-access places, are to be sampled then an extension hose is also required.

There are two basic types of suction pump available, the bellows type as shown in Fig. 2.12 or a piston type as shown in Fig. 2.4. Each pump is designed to pass a measured volume of air for an operating stroke, the bellows type passing 100 ml and the piston type having two possibilities: namely a full stroke at 100 ml and a half stroke at 50 ml. Thus it is important to ensure that the correct tube is used with the pump for which it is designed.

The type of detector tube available depends upon the gas to be measured. This dictates the chemical reaction that occurs within the tube in order to produce the indicating stain. With some types the concentration is indicated by means of the length of a coloured stain measured against a single scale inscribed on the glass wall of the tube, whereas a double scale is provided on some to accommodate two different numbers of pump stroke. Indication of concentration may also be by colour change rather than length of stain; a means for colour comparison is available either built into the tube or as a separate item.

The construction of the tubes also varies for different gases depending upon the chemical reaction producing the stain. For example, it may be necessary to activate the tube by breaking an ampoule of reagent within the tube as shown in Fig. 2.13, this ampoule containing either dry powder, a liquid or a vapour. Alternatively, it may be necessary to employ a pre-tube before the indicator thus placing the two tubes in tandem with a short connection between them. Instruction on the method of use is given in a leaflet enclosed with the box of tubes.

Method

Using the bellows pump

Before making a test it is necessary to undertake some preliminary checks on the pump.

1   Check for a leak in the bellows: without breaking the ends of the glass detector tube insert it into the pump orifice and squeeze the bellows to close and release immediately. If the bellows remain closed then no leaks exist; a leaking pump would open during the test.

2   Check for a blockage in the suction channels: squeeze the bellows to close and with no tube in position the bellows should spring open immediately on release. If the channels are blocked the bellows would open relatively slowly.

Note: to undertake the test read the instructions supplied with the box of detector tubes.

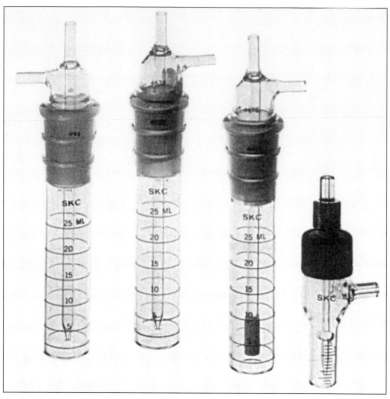

Fig. 2.11. Typical impingers (SKC Ltd).

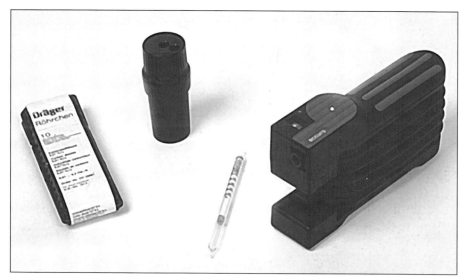

Fig. 2.12. Bellows type pump for colorimetric detector (Dräger Ltd).

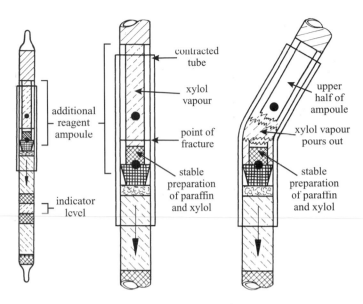

additional
reagent
ampoule

indicator
level

contracted
tube

xylol
vapour

point of
fracture

stable
preparation
of paraffin
and xylol

upper
half of
ampoule

xylol vapour
pours out

stable
preparation
of paraffin
and xylol

Fig. 2.13. Detector tube with ampoule (Dräger Ltd).

3 Break both glass end seals on the detector tube using the tip breaking device. If an internal ampoule is provided, break that as per instructions.

4 Insert the tube into the suction orifice of the pump making sure the arrow on the tube points towards the pump. If a pre-tube is required, break its seals and connect it to the assembly according to the instructions.

5 Squeeze the bellows and release immediately. They will open at a rate governed by the flow resistance of the tube. Do not hinder this operation by trying to control the rate of opening. If sufficient gas is present in the air sampled a dark stain will appear from the zero and extend up the tube in response to the concentration of the gas present (Fig. 2.14).

6 If the scale on the tube requires one stroke then read the indicated concentration corresponding to the end of the stain, as inscribed on the wall of the tube.

7 If the scale requires more pump strokes repeat operation 5, carefully counting the number of strokes until the required number is reached. The range of some tubes can be extended by increasing the number of strokes but this must be done according to the maker's instructions. A stroke counter is fitted to the latest pumps. At the end of the test read the concentration as described above.

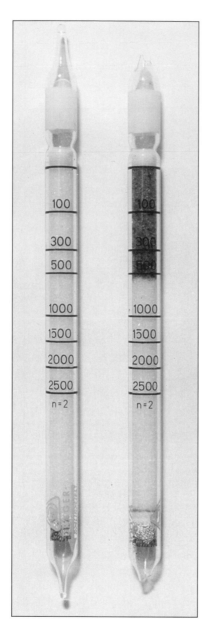

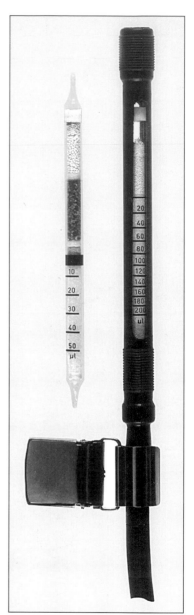

Fig. 2.14. *(left)*   Used and unused detector tubes showing stain.

Fig. 2.15. *(right)*   Long-term detector tube in holder (Casella Ltd).

Using the piston pump

Before making the test it is necessary to undertake some preliminary checks on the pump.

1   Check the valves for leakage: without breaking the ends of the glass detector tube insert it into the pump orifice, move the pump handle so that the two red dots are not in line and pull out the handle several times fully quite quickly, then pull out the handle just 6 mm, hold for two minutes and release. If the handle returns to within 1.5 mm of the closed position the valves are in order. If not the valves require to be lubricated according to the manufacturer's instructions.

2   Check the field volume: insert an unbroken tube as before, align the red dots and pull out the handle fully until it locks in the open position, wait for one minute then twist the handle a quarter turn to release it. If it is in order it should return to within 6 mm (3 inch) or less of the fully closed position, but do not allow it to spring back but guide it gently as it returns. If it does not return as described lubrication is required as instructed by the manufacturer.

Note: to undertake the test read the instructions supplied with the box of detector tubes.

3   Break both glass seals on the detector tube using the tip breaking orifice provided on the pump.

4   Insert the tube into the pump making sure that the arrow on the tube is pointing towards the pump. If twin tubes are used connect the ends marked with a 'C' by means of a short length of rubber tubing.

5   Push the pump handle fully in, align the red dots and pull out to the desired stroke position either half way or fully out according to the requirements of the test as instructed by the makers. The handle will lock in position and not return. If sufficient gas is present in the air sampled a dark stain will appear from the zero end extending up the tube in response to the gas concentration present. Do not release the handle until the stain has stopped extending.

6   The concentration can be read as that inscribed on the wall of the detector tube corresponding to the end of the stain.

7   If the tube requires more strokes of the pump as indicated by the makers in the instructions sheet, then twist the handle one quarter of a turn to release the locked position and repeat operation 5 for the required number of strokes. Carefully note the number of strokes. Read the concentration as instructed.

To measure the long-term time-weighted average concentration of a gas using a colorimetric detector tube

The gases listed below can be detected over a period up to 4 hours using specifically designed long-running or long-term detector tubes by Dräger, as shown in their current handbook.

Acetic acid	Hydrocyanic acid
Acetone	Hydrogen fluoride
Ammonia	Hydrogen sulphide
Benzene	Methylene chloride
Carbon dioxide	Nitrogen dioxide
Carbon disulphide	Nitrous fumes
Carbon monoxide	Perchloroethylene
Chlorine	Sulphur dioxide
Ethanol	Toluene
Hydrocarbon	Trichloroethylene
Hydrochloric acid	Vinyl chloride

Equipment required

A low flow sampling pump capable of a constant flow rate of 15–20 ml min^{-1} but preferably the peristaltic pump made by Dräger, rubber tubing incorporating a long running tube holder (Fig. 2.15), a calibrated flowmeter or a soap bubble device.

Method

1   Check the pump for leaks.
2   Break off the ends of the glass Dräger tube.
3   Place the tube in the holder making sure the arrows point towards the pump and connect the tubing to the pump.
4   Start the pump and check and adjust the flow rate to between 15 and 20 ml min^{-1}, noting the time of start.
5   Run the pump for no more than 4 hours, noting the time when switched off.
6   Read the length of stain on the Dräger tube noting the number of μl indicated.
7   Calculate the amount of air passed through the pump in litres during the sampling period by multiplying the number of minutes of sampling by the flow rate in litres per minute (*V*).

The time-weighted average airborne concentration in parts 10^{-6} (ppm) is calculated as follows:

$$\text{Concentration} = \frac{\text{indicated μl of gas}}{V} \text{ ppm}$$

General

The manufacturers of detector tubes publish comprehensive handbooks outlining the main features of all their tubes and give guidance on where inaccuracies could occur. There are some important general remarks that should be made with regard to detector tube sampling in order to guide the user and to ensure that the results obtained are seen in perspective:

1   The results obtained for a specific gas can be considered reliable provided that no other gas is present that could interfere with the chemical reaction taking place inside the tube to produce the stain. The handbooks refer to interference gases. Therefore it is important that no test is undertaken without consulting the handbook.

2   The pump must be in good condition with a good seal between the tube and the pump suction orifice.

3   The tubes must be not more than 2 years old and preferably should be stored in a domestic-type refrigerator. Dates are given on the box.

4   Detector tubes are designed to operate at 20 °C and normal atmospheric pressure (1013 mb, 760 mmHg) and 50% relative humidity. In most cases a wide range of variation from these conditions can be tolerated but where tubes are sensitive to these factors correction charts are provided in the box supplied.

5   It is important to use a fresh tube for each test. If no stain appears after a test that tube must be discarded and not re-used.

Further reading

American Conference of Governmental Industrial Hygienists (1995) *Air Sampling Instruments*, 8th edn. ACGIH, Cincinnati.

American Conference of Governmental Industrial Hygienists (1997) *NIOHS Manual of Analytical Methods*, 4th edn. ACGIH, Cincinnati.

Brown, R.H. (1995) The sampling of gases and vapours: principles and methods. In: *Occupational Hygiene* (eds J.M. Harrington & K. Gardiner), pp. 84–98. Blackwell Science, Oxford.

Dragerwerk AG (1997) *Dräger Tube Handbook*. Dräger Limited, Blyth.

Health and Safety Executive (1998) *Occupational Exposure Limits*, Guidance Note EH40/year. HMSO, London.

SI 1999 No. 437 and Approved Code of Practice (1999) *Control of Substances Hazardous to Health Regulations*. HMSO, London.

Thain, W. (1980) *Monitoring Toxic Gases in the Atmosphere for Hygiene and Pollution Control*. Pergamon Press, Oxford.

3 Heat

Introduction

The human body generates heat as a result of the burning of fuel in the form of food metabolism. If that heat is dissipated too slowly deep body temperatures will rise, the opposite occurring if the outward heat flow is too fast. The rate of heat transfer between the body and its surroundings depends upon the thermal environment in contact with the skin. In order to effect a heat exchange between the two environments, that is, inside and outside the body, the normal heat transfer mechanisms of conduction, convection, evaporation and radiation take place. Of these, convection and evaporation are inter-related and play a major role in dissipating body heat, therefore the temperature and the moisture content of the air are important parameters to measure. This is done by taking the wet and dry bulb temperatures of the air in the workplace. The study of the relationship between air temperature and moisture content is called 'psychrometry', that is the study of the behaviour of dry air and water vapour mixtures. Some further details on this topic are given later.

The radiant heat exchange between a person and the surroundings also plays an important part in the regulation of body heat flow as the skin radiates heat to colder surfaces and receives radiant heat from hotter surfaces. The rate of radiant heat flow is proportional to the difference between the fourth power of the absolute temperatures of the surfaces exchanging heat. The exact equation for the human body and its surroundings is difficult to establish because there are many surfaces at different temperatures, of different emissivities and subtending different solid angles to the body surfaces, which, in turn, are constantly changing as the person moves. To integrate all these, the concept of 'mean radiant temperature' is used. This is defined as the hypothetical temperature of a uniform black enclosure that exchanges the same amount of heat with the body as the non-uniform enclosure. The globe thermometer can provide a good indication of the radiant heat exchange likely to be found at a point although it is affected by air velocity and therefore does not provide the true mean radiant temperature unless adjusted for air velocity.

Rates of heat convection and evaporation are also affected by the movement of air around the body, therefore it is important to measure the air speed at a workplace. Thus the four parameters that must be tested to obtain a true indication of the thermal environment are: dry bulb, wet bulb and globe temperatures, and the air velocity.

When any one or more of these parameters is excessive the heat flow to or from the body will be out of balance, resulting in an uncomfortable or stressful situation. Many indoor workplaces display unsatisfactory thermal environmental conditions. For example, high radiant sources can be found in steelworks and glass making, high humidities in laundries, kitchens and deep wet mines, and cold conditions in deep-freeze stores and warehouses. Extremes of heat and cold are experienced at some time of the year in many outdoor work stations with regard to radiant heat, hot and cold air temperature, high and low humidities and high winds.

Whilst no legal standards exist in the United Kingdom for a satisfactory or safe thermal environment, there is a duty described under the Workplace Health, Safety and Welfare Regulations. Regulation 7 states: 'During working hours, the temperature in all workplaces inside buildings shall be reasonable'.

Equipment available

Dry bulb thermometers

These are normally mercury in glass thermometers with a variety of ranges to suit the environment to be measured. A useful range for indoor work is 5 ° to 65 °C, and for most outdoor work stations in Great Britain −15 ° to 40 °C. The small thermometers (scale length 100 mm) measure to 0.5 °C, having scale divisions of that order, but the larger instruments (scale length 175 mm) can be read to increments of 0.1 °C although they are usually marked with the same divisions as the smaller ones.

There are also a variety of electrical thermometers available using either: thermocouple, diode or platinum resistance principles with analogue or digital read-out.

Wet bulb thermometers

These are simply dry bulb instruments as described above but with the bulb covered in a clean cotton wick wetted with distilled water. As the water evaporates from the wick, heat will be removed from the bulb thus reducing the indicated temperature to below that of the dry bulb unless the air is fully saturated with water vapour and none can evaporate. The bulb can either be ventilated by an induced air current or it can rely upon natural air currents to remove the evaporated water vapour. In the latter case the reading on the scale is referred to as the 'natural wet bulb temperature'.

It is also possible to fit a wetted wick to certain electrical temperature indicators.

Sling psychrometer (whirling hygrometer)

This consists of wet and dry bulb thermometers mounted in a frame with a swivel at the top end so that it can be rotated by hand to induce an air current to flow over the bulbs. Most instruments have a distilled water reservoir into which the wick covering the wet bulb dips to provide a continuous flow of water (Fig. 3.1). Relative humidity can be obtained from the readings of this device either by using a chart supplied with the instrument or by using a psychrometric chart (see Fig. 3.9).

Aspirated psychrometer

This is a larger but more precise instrument consisting of wet and dry bulb thermometers mounted in a frame arranged so that air is induced to flow over the bulbs at a regulated rate by means of a fan powered by a clockwork or electric motor. The wick is not continuously wetted but has to be dipped into a separate container of distilled water before a reading is taken. The bulbs of the thermometers are shielded from radiant heat by tubes that act as entry ports

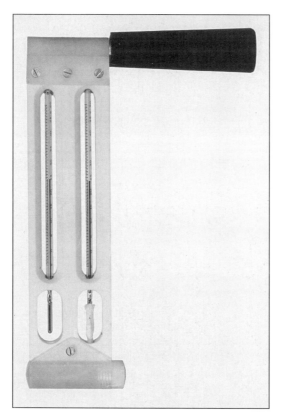 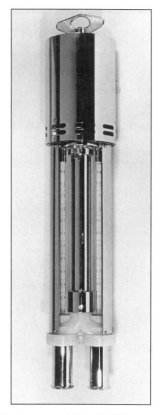

Fig. 3.1. *(left)*   Sling psychrometer (whirling hygrometer) (Casella Ltd).

Fig. 3.2. *(right)*   Aspirated psychrometer (Casella Ltd).

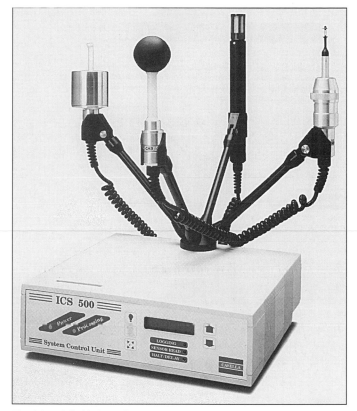

Fig. 3.3. Digital indoor climate meter (Casella Ltd).

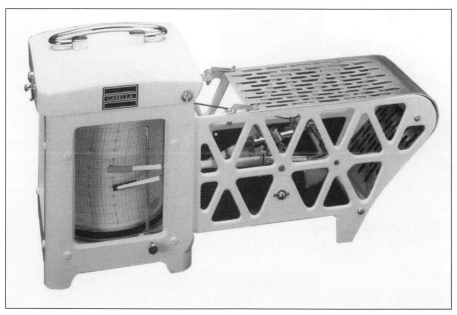

Fig. 3.4. Thermal hydrograph (Casella Ltd).

guiding the air at a speed of between 3.5 and 5.0 m s^{-1} (Fig. 3.2). Relative humidity is obtained as with the sling psychrometer described above.

Continuous recording of temperature and humidity
The thermohygrograph is the traditional instrument for continuously recording values of temperature and humidity. The temperature is sensed by a bi-metallic strip whose curvature changes with temperature. The humidity is sensed by an element consisting of strands of human hair whose length changes with humidity. Both elements are connected via magnifying linkages to recording pens, which scribe lines on a paper-covered, clockwork-driven, rotating drum. These elegant instruments have been popular as functional display pieces for years (Fig. 3.4). The recording period can be either daily, weekly or monthly depending upon the rotating speed of the drum, replaceable paper charts being available for the three periods. With the hair-type humidity sensing element there is a loss of precision at the ends of the scale.

For more precise work some of the latest electronic instruments can be coupled to chart or digital recorders.

Globe thermometer
A mercury in glass thermometer is placed with its bulb in the centre of a matt black sphere or globe. The diameters of the globes available are usually 150 mm or 44 mm (Fig. 3.5). The larger globe takes approximately 20 minutes to reach equilibrium with its surroundings but the smaller one is quicker. Most of the published thermal standards are based upon research using the larger globe thermometer, therefore, in spite of its slow response time, this size is to be preferred.

Kata thermometer
This is an alcohol in glass thermometer having a large silvered bulb at its base and a small bulb at the top of the stem (Fig. 3.6), which is inscribed with marks on the top and bottom corresponding to a temperature difference of 3 °C. They are available in three ranges: 38–35 °C, 54.5–51.5 °C and 65.5–62.5 °C. Also inscribed on the stem is a number known as the Kata Factor, which is specific to each instrument. The device is used to determine the cooling power of the air by timing the rate of fall of the liquid by contraction between the two marks having first heated the lower bulb to expand the liquid up the stem. From this the air velocity can be calculated or determined from a chart supplied with the instrument. The Kata thermometer is particularly useful in measuring air velocities below the range of most air flow meters, i.e. less than 0.5 m s^{-1}.

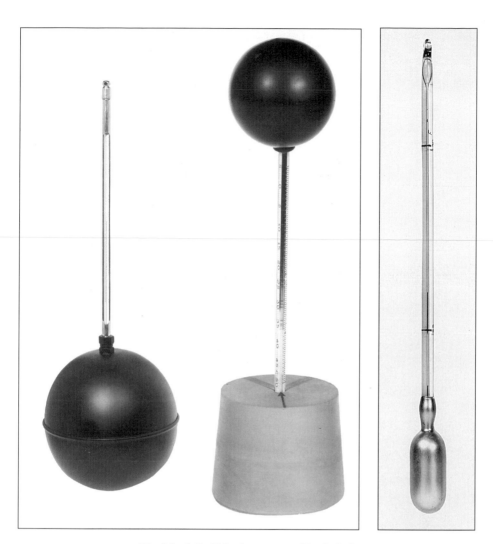

Fig. 3.5. *(left)* Globe thermometers (Casella Ltd).

Fig. 3.6. *(right)* Kata thermometer (Casella Ltd).

Integrating instruments

In order to obtain a single index from wet bulb, dry bulb, globe temperatures and air velocity, instruments are available that measure these parameters electrically and integrate the results into a single value. This is in addition to having the facility to indicate the individual values in turn by means of a selector switch (Fig. 3.3. and 3.7). As with any instrument that provides a reading on a meter it requires to be calibrated from time to time against accurate mercury in glass thermometers in an environmental chamber.

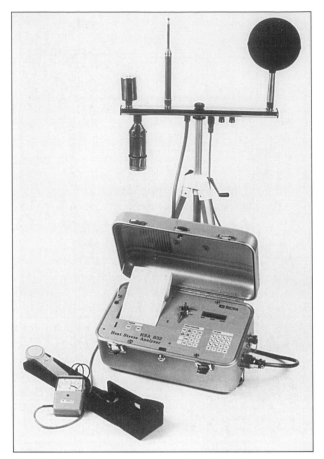

Fig. 3.7. Integrating heat stress meter (Shaw City Ltd).

There is an instrument known as a 'Botsball thermometer', which consists of a globe thermometer where the complete globe section is covered with a black wetted wick. With such a device all four parameters mentioned earlier act upon the globe producing a temperature that approximates to the heat index known as the WBGT (wet bulb globe temperature).

There is also an indoor climate monitor, which, in addition to measuring and integrating the four main thermal parameters, can be adapted to detect and indicate levels of various gases (such as CO_2, CO, O_3) plus airborne dust concentrations. Up to eight parameters may be monitored simultaneously and fourteen derived parameters recorded. The whole instrument uses fully integrated Windows™ software (Fig. 3.3). This instrument is particularly valuable in investigating suspected 'sick buildings', where not only thermal conditions but also the above gases, amongst others, may be implicated.

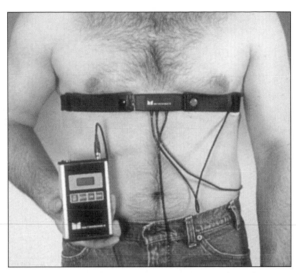

Fig. 3.8. Metrosonics heat stress monitor (Shaw City Ltd).

Heat stress monitor

In addition to monitoring the working environment it is possible to monitor the worker using a portable heat stress monitor. This consists of a miniature data logger that receives signals from various sensors attached to an employee's body by means of an elastic belt. Heart rate and temperature are sensed from which a Strain index is calculated and indicated with audible signals when the index reaches a warning level and an action level. The device can be set for three age ranges of worker (under 36, 36–50 and over 50 years) and for two levels of clothing: single layer (work clothes or cotton overalls) and multiple layer (double cotton or impermeable coveralls). The instrument is illustrated in Fig. 3.8.

To use the psychrometric chart

The driving force that makes water evaporate is the difference in 'vapour pressure' between the air and the water surface. The maximum vapour pressure that can occur at any temperature is known as the 'saturation vapour pressure' and this varies with temperature according to the 100% saturation curve on the psychrometric chart shown in Fig. 3.9. The vapour pressure and moisture content lines are in the same position on the chart. Curves of relative humidity (percentage saturation) of below 100% are shown lying under this curve in increments of 10% with the dry bulb temperature as the base line and wet bulbs at an oblique angle. Other information shown is moisture content, specific enthalpy and specific volume. This latter unit is the reciprocal of the density of the air and water vapour mixture.

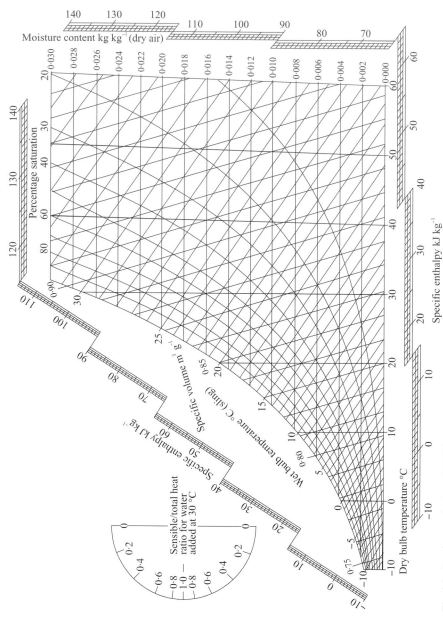

Fig. 3.9. Psychrometric chart (CIBSE).

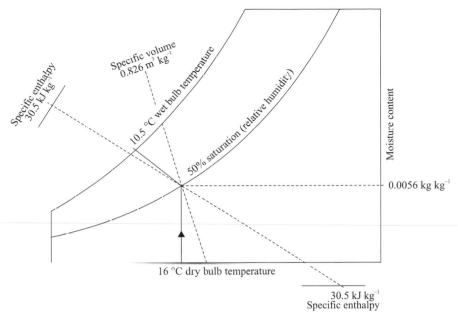

Fig. 3.10. Diagram to illustrate use of psychrometric chart.

To use this chart it is necessary to measure the wet and dry bulb temperature at a workplace. The point showing the conditions in the workroom air is at the intersection of the lines representing these two values on the chart. All other values can be read by extending lines across the appropriate scales as shown in the example on the sketch in Fig. 3.10.

Example
A sling psychrometer measured the wet and dry bulb temperatures to be 10.5 °C and 16 °C respectively. From the chart in Fig. 3.9 the following values can be obtained as indicated by the broken lines in Fig. 3.10:

Relative humidity (percentage saturation):	50%
Moisture content:	0.0056 kg kg^{-1} (i.e. kg of water vapour per kg of dry air)
Specific enthalpy:	30.5 kJ kg^{-1} of dry air
Specific volume:	0. 826 m^3 kg^{-1}
Air density (reciprocal of specific volume):	1.21 kg m^{-3}
Vapour pressure:	8.7 mb

(vapour pressure in mb can be obtained by multiplying moisture content in kg kg^{-1} by 1560).

Heat indices

Many scientists have tried to combine all or most of the parameters mentioned previously together with the work rate and clothing worn into a single index, which would give an indication of the degree of discomfort or stress to he expected of that environment. Many indices have been devised to suit a particular industry. Each index emphasises some factors more than others and thus may not be ideal for the specific problem under consideration. The index that is covered in the American Conference of Government Industrial Hygienists (ACGIH) list of threshold limit values is the WBGT. Given with this index is a table showing maximum values for various work rates together with recommended work and rest periods. An example calculation is given in the following section with Table 3.2 showing WBGT values, as published by the ACGIH (see page 75). Other heat indices are given in Figs 3.19–3.21.

Where heat loss is concerned, as with outdoor situations when temperatures are low and wind speeds are high, the wind chill factor chart should be used as shown in Fig. 3.23. With this factor only dry bulb temperature and air velocity are significant.

The measurement of the thermal environment

Aim

It is often necessary to examine the thermal load imposed upon employees in hot or cold industries or in workplaces out of doors in hot or cold climates. By measuring four parameters – wet and dry bulb temperature, air velocity and globe temperature – heat stress indices can be obtained and the thermal components making up the workplace environment evaluated so that the more extreme factors can be improved to the benefit of the worker.

Equipment required

Kata thermometer, two mercury in glass thermometers of the correct range to suit the environment to be measured, a globe thermometer, stop-watch, thermos flask, sling psychrometer, tissues, 25 ml beaker, muslin wick, distilled water, rubber bung bored out to take one of the thermometers, aluminium foil, string, scissors, metal polish and soft cloth and a tripod stand with clamps.

Method

1　Before starting the survey fill the thermos flask with very hot or boiling water.
2　Polish the bulb of the Kata thermometer and record the Kata Factor inscribed on the stem of the instrument.

3   To prepare the dry bulb thermometer, carefully fit the rubber bung to the lower end and attach a piece of aluminium foil round the bung to shield the bulb of the thermometer but not to restrict any air flow around it. The foil should be fitted shiny side out.

4   To prepare the natural wet bulb, attach the muslin wick over the bulb of the other thermometer, covering it completely. Wet the wick with distilled water and allow the loose end of the wick to dip into the beaker containing distilled water. Hang the beaker just below the bulb by means of string or sticky tape, ensuring that it is clear of the bulb in order to allow unrestricted air flow.

5   Check that the bulb of the globe thermometer is in the centre of the globe.

6   Arrange these instruments on the tripod stand as shown in Fig. 3.11 and place at the workplace to be measured, making sure that the sensors are situated in the vicinity of the worker's head during normal operations.

7   Allow about 20 minutes for the instruments to reach equilibrium and record the values of dry bulb, natural wet bulb and globe temperatures.

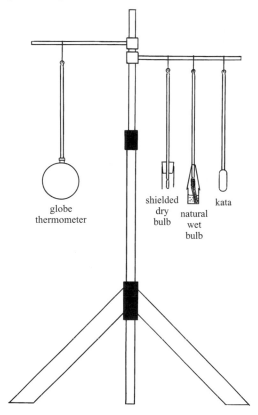

Fig. 3.11. Arrangement of thermometers on a stand.

8   Measure the air velocity using the Kata thermometer as
follows: Immerse the bulb of the Kata thermometer in the hot
water in the thermos flask and when the alcohol column reaches
the upper bulb remove it immediately. Make sure that there is a
continuous column of alcohol between the two bulbs as
sometimes a vapour lock occurs, which disappears if the bulb is
further heated. Do not over-heat the bulb as the thermometer may
burst. Wipe the silvered bulb dry and using a stop-watch time the
fall of the alcohol column between the two marks on the stem of
the thermometer. Repeat the process three or four times, noting
the times, and calculate the mean.

9   Measure the air humidity by using the sling psychrometer.
Make sure that the wick is wetted and the reservoir is full of
distilled water and that the loose end of the wick reaches the
water. Hold the instrument by the handle and rotate it as fast as
possible to allow air to flow over the bulbs for at least one
minute. Read the wet bulb first and record both temperatures.
This should be repeated several times until the temperatures taken
are consistently the same. Evaluate the relative humidity from the
chart provided with the instrument or by using the psychrometric
chart. Ensure that parts of the body are well away from the bulbs
when reading these instruments.

Results and calculations

The results should be recorded as they are taken on a table similar to
Table 3.1. The air velocity can be calculated from the Kata thermometer results as follows:

$$v = \left\{ \frac{1}{b}\left(\frac{H}{\theta} - a\right) \right\}^2 \left(\text{from } H = \theta\left(a + b\sqrt{v}\right)\right)$$

where

$\qquad H \;$ = cooling power = Kata Factor ÷ cooling time in
$\qquad\qquad$ seconds

$\qquad \theta \;$ = mean Kata range – dry bulb temperature

a and $b \;$ = constants for the instrument, and

$\qquad v \;$ = air velocity.

Alternatively, use the chart supplied with the instrument. Three
examples are given in Figs 3.12–3.14, with the broken lines representing a worked example.

   The mean radiant temperature can be calculated from:

$$\left(T_r\right)^4\left(10^{-9}\right) = \left(T_g\right)^4\left(10^{-9}\right) + 0.247\sqrt{v\left(t_g - t\right)}$$

where

$T_r = 273 + t_r$

t_r = mean radiant temperature °C

$T_g = 273 + t_g$, and

t_g = globe temperature reading in °C

The WBGT can be calculated from:

for indoor use, $\text{WBGT} = 0.7t'_n + 0.3t_g$

for outdoor use, $\text{WBGT} = 0.7t'_n + 0.2t_g + 0.1t$

where

t'_n = natural wet bulb temperature °C

t_g = globe temperature °C, and

t = dry bulb temperature °C

Note that the ventilated wet bulb can be used in place of the natural wet bulb according to the following rules:

• if the relative humidity of the air is below 25%, add 1 °C to the ventilated wet bulb temperature;

Table 3.1. Suggested layout for a thermal survey results sheet

Survey. . . . . Date						
Location . . . . Measured by						
Measuring station			Readings				Mean
			1	2	3	4	5	
	Time							
	Dry bulb (*t*)							
	Natural wet bulb (*t′*n)							
	Globe (*t*g)							
	Sling or aspirated	wet bulb (*t′*)						
		dry bulb (*t*)						
	Relative humidity (%)							
	Kata factor Mean temperature range							
	Cooling time (s)							
	Air velocity (*v*)							
	Mean radiant temperature (*t*r)							
	WBGT							

- if the relative humidity of the air is between 25 and 50%, add 0.5 °C to the ventilated wet bulb temperature;

- if the relative humidity of the air is above 50%, use the ventilated wet bulb temperature.

In order to evaluate this index it is necessary to establish the work rate of the person whose workplace is being measured, that is, as light, moderate, or heavy. Some examples are given as follows:

Light work rate: sitting, standing with small hand movements. Examples: desk work or light assembly work.

Moderate work rate: walking, standing with heavy hand or light arm work. Examples: supervisory work covering a wide area, messenger work, bench work with heavier items, press operation.

Heavy work rate: standing with heavy arm work, work involving whole body. Examples: sawing and filing, lifting from floor, shovelling, walking carrying loads, pulling or pushing trolleys or barrows, climbing ladders or steep steps most of the time.

Using Table 3.2 the recommended maximum WBGT can be established for different work rates.

Other heat indices can be obtained by reference to some of the publications given in the further reading section at the end of this chapter.

Possible problems

1 The Kata bulb may be dirty and this will increase the cooling time and provide an exaggeratedly low air velocity result.
2 Dirty wicks or the use of non-distilled water on the wet bulbs will result in a lowered evaporation rate giving an exaggeratedly high humidity.
3 When reading thermometers make sure that no other heat source such as human hands or breath comes into contact with them.
4 Ventilated wet bulbs will immediately rise in temperature when the ventilation ceases. They must therefore be read quickly to prevent a falsely high humidity being derived.
5 When undertaking an indoor survey it is useful to note the outdoor conditions with regard to temperature, moisture content and wind velocity as these factors can have an important effect on indoor values.

Table 3.2. Maximum values for work rates and recommended work/rest regimes

Work/rest regime	Total work load		
	Light	Medium	Heavy
Continuous work	30.0	26.7	25.0
75% work, 25% rest	30.6	28.0	25.9
50% work, 50% rest	31.4	29.4	27.9
25% work, 75% rest	32.2	31.1	30.0

The use of the Kata thermometer chart
(Figs 3.12–3.14)

Example: Kata Factor (cooling factor) 539, temperature range 38–35 °C mean cooling time as measured 95 s, and air temperature (dry bulb) 18 °C.

Procedure
1 Draw a line (A) to join 539 on 'cooling factor' scale with the measured mean cooling time 95 s on 'cooling time' scale and extend it to intersect with the 'cooling power' scale (in this example cooling power = 5.7).
2 From that point on 'cooling power' scale draw a line (B) to join with 18 °C on the 'temperature' line and extend it to intersect with the 'air speed' scale.
3 Air speed can be read in either m s^{-1} or ft min^{-1} (in this example air velocity is shown to be 0.26 m s^{-1}).

The use of the globe thermometer chart
(Figs 3.15–3.18)

Example: globe temperature (t_g) 22 °C, air temperature (dry bulb) (t) 18 °C, and air velocity from Kata (v) 0.26 m s^{-1}.

Procedure
1 Subtract $t_g - t$ (22 − 18 = + 4) and join $t_g - t$ (+ 4) on scale A to velocity (0.26) on scale B and extend to cut scale C (line 1). In the example it gives a value of + 0.5 on scale C.
2 Join that point on scale C (+ 0.5) with t_g (22 °C) on scale D (line 2).
3 The mean radiant temperature can be read from the point where line 2 crosses scale E (mean temperature of the surroundings). In this example it reads 26.8 °C.

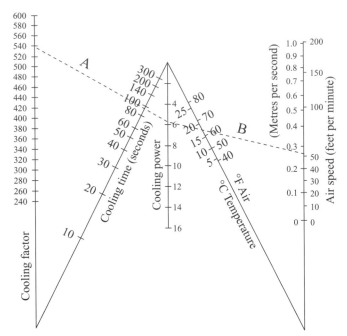

Fig. 3.12. Kata thermometer chart for temperature range 38–35 °C (Casella Ltd).

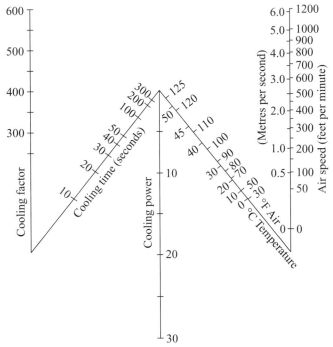

Fig. 3.13. Kata thermometer chart for temperature range 54.5–51.5 °C (Casella Ltd).

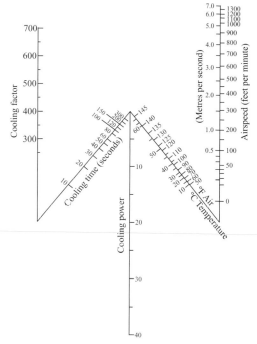

Fig. 3.14. Kata thermometer chart for temperature range 65.5–62.5 °C (Casella Ltd).

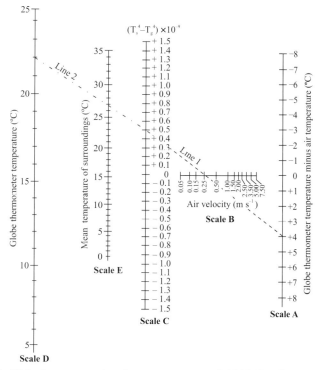

Fig. 3.15. Globe thermometer chart for temperature range 5–25 °C (Casella Ltd).

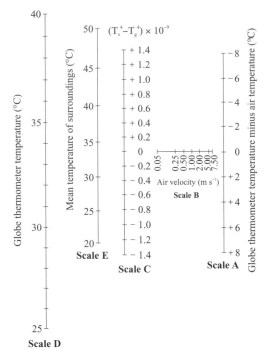

Fig. 3.16. Globe thermometer chart for temperature range 5–25 °C (Casella Ltd).

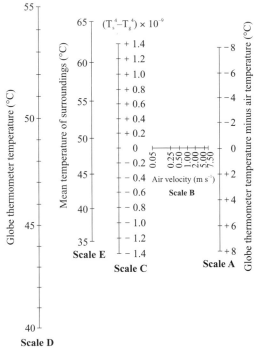

Fig. 3.17. Globe thermometer chart for temperature range 40–55 °C (Casella Ltd).

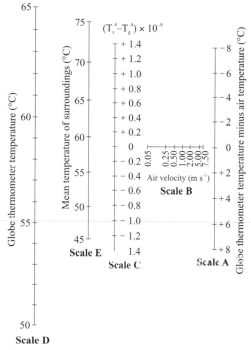

Fig. 3.18. Globe thermometer chart for temperature range 50–65 °C (Casella Ltd).

To use the normal scale of corrected effective temperature (Fig. 3.20)

Measure wet bulb, globe temperatures and air velocity as described above. For the purposes of this example the following temperatures were measured: globe 32 °C, wet bulb 27 °C, air velocity 0.5 m s^{-1}.

Procedure

1   On the chart draw a line joining the wet bulb temperature with the globe (or dry bulb if globe is not used).

2   Where this line crosses the air velocity line the normal corrected effective temperature can be read off as 28 °C from the main body of the chart.

3   Where a correction for work rate is made (in this example a work rate of 204 W m^{-2} is used) produce a line from the intersection with the air velocity up the work rate extension to the chart until it intersects with the 204 line. The normal corrected effective temperature adjusted for work rate is read as 33 °C.

Air velocity

ft min^{-1}	m s^{-1}	m s^{-1} plotted	m s^{-1} error
20	0.1016	0.100	0.0016
100	0.508	0.500	0.008
200	1.015	1.000	0.016
300	1.524	1.500	0.024
400	2.032	2.000	0.032
500	2.540	2.500	0.040
600	3.048	3.000	0.048
700	3.556	3.500	0.056

Conversion factor
ft min^{-1} × 0.00508 = m s^{-1}
Factor used
ft min^{-1} × 0.005 (error 1.6%)

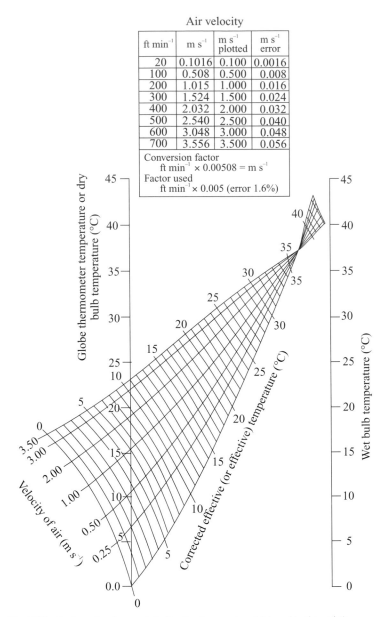

Fig. 3.19. Basic scale of corrected effective temperature (stripped to the waist).

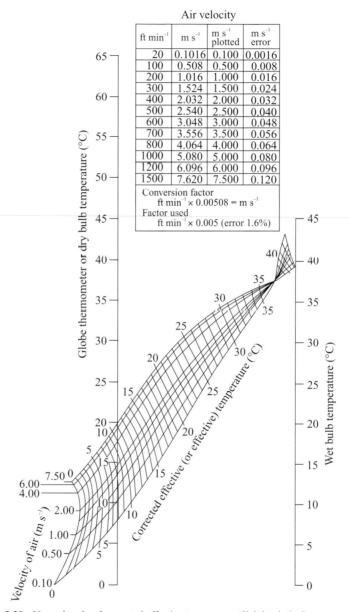

Air velocity

ft min^{-1}	m s^{-1}	m s^{-1} plotted	m s^{-1} error
20	0.1016	0.100	0.0016
100	0.508	0.500	0.008
200	1.016	1.000	0.016
300	1.524	1.500	0.024
400	2.032	2.000	0.032
500	2.540	2.500	0.040
600	3.048	3.000	0.048
700	3.556	3.500	0.056
800	4.064	4.000	0.064
1000	5.080	5.000	0.080
1200	6.096	6.000	0.096
1500	7.620	7.500	0.120

Conversion factor
  ft min^{-1} × 0.00508 = m s^{-1}
Factor used
  ft min^{-1} × 0.005 (error 1.6%)

Fig. 3.20. Normal scale of corrected effective temperature (lightly clothed).

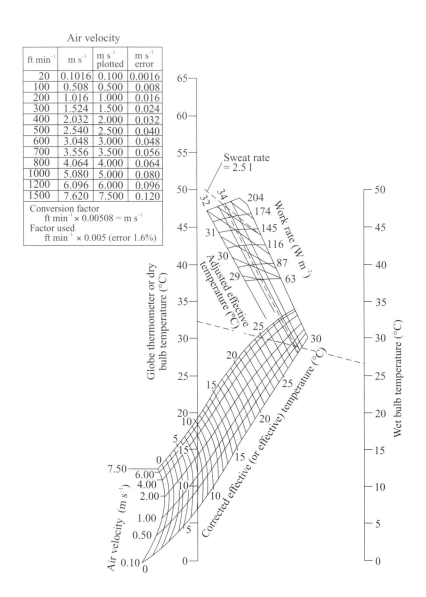

Air velocity

ft min⁻¹	m s⁻¹	m s⁻¹ plotted	m s⁻¹ error
20	0.1016	0.100	0.0016
100	0.508	0.500	0.008
200	1.016	1.000	0.016
300	1.524	1.500	0.024
400	2.032	2.000	0.032
500	2.540	2.500	0.040
600	3.048	3.000	0.048
700	3.556	3.500	0.056
800	4.064	4.000	0.064
1000	5.080	5.000	0.080
1200	6.096	6.000	0.096
1500	7.620	7.500	0.120

Conversion factor
  ft min⁻¹ × 0.00508 = m s⁻¹
Factor used
  ft min⁻¹ × 0.005 (error 1.6%)

Fig. 3.21. Normal scale of corrected effective temperature (lightly clothed) with additional nomogram including work rate.

To obtain wind chill factor using chart

Wind chill is a function of air dry bulb temperature and air velocity only. That is it represents the worst case where there is no radiant heat gain component, and moisture content will be low because of the limited water-holding capacity of low temperature air even if it is saturated.

Procedure

1   Measure the dry bulb temperature and air velocity at the occupied site. Note, if measuring outdoor conditions the wind direction is unlikely to be steady, therefore a non-directional air velocity meter should be used such as a cup anemometer (Fig. 3.22).

2   On the wind chill chart (Fig. 3.23) draw a vertical line through the dry bulb temperature and a horizontal line through the air velocity. The intersection of these two lines represents the condition measured.

3   The curved lines on the chart represent lines of equal bodily heat loss, or cooling effect in W m^{-2}. Follow the curved line that passes through the measured condition until it reaches the line of zero velocity. If no printed line passes through the point, draw an imaginary line parallel to the one closest to it until it reaches the zero velocity line. The wind chill factor is read as the dry bulb temperature at this point.

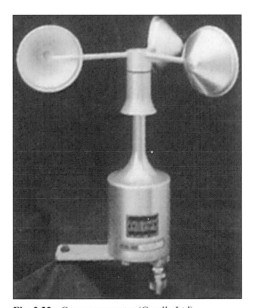

Fig. 3.22. Cup anemometer (Casella Ltd).

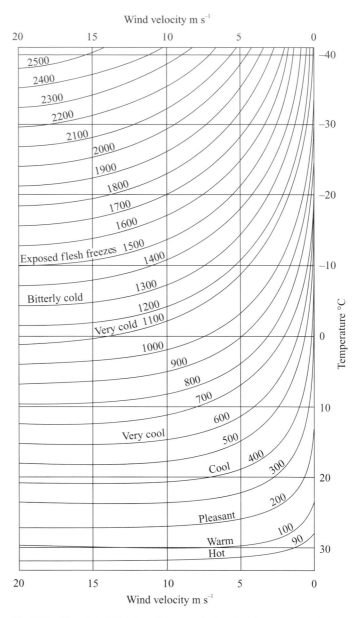

Fig. 3.23. The wind chill index. Values marked against the curves are the rate of cooling in kcal m^{-2} h^{-1} (multiply by 1.16 to convert to W m^{-2}) at different wind velocities (m s^{-1}) and temperature (°C).

Example

Find the wind chill factor corresponding to a measured dry bulb temperature 0 °C at a wind speed of 5 m s^{-1}.

The intersection of these two lines occurs at the cooling power line of 1050 W m^{-2}. The curved line passing through this condition intersects the zero velocity line at −25 °C, which is the wind chill factor for this condition.

Further reading

BOHS (1990) *The Thermal Environment*, Technical Guide No. 8. Science Reviews, Leeds.

Chartered Institute of Building Services Engineers Guide, Section CI/2. Pads of 50 charts sized A3 suitable for permanent records are available from CIBSE (for address see Appendix II).

Fanger, P.O. (1970) Thermal comfort. In: *Analysis and Application in Environmental Engineering* (ed. P.O. Fanger). McGraw-Hill, Maidenhead.

Gill, F.S. (1980) Heat. In: *Occupational Hygiene* (eds H.A. Waldron & J.M. Harrington), pp. 225–256. Blackwell Scientific Publications, Oxford.

Harrington, J.M., Gill, F.S., Aw, T.C. & Gardiner, K. (1998) *Pocket Consultant in Occupational Health*. Blackwell Science, Oxford.

Kerslake, D M K (1972) *The Stress of Hot Environments*. Cambridge University Press, Cambridge.

Parsons, K.C. (1993) *Human Thermal Environments*. Taylor and Francis, London.

SI 1992 2051 and Approved Code of Practice (1992) *Workplace Health Safety and Welfare Regulations 1992*. HMSO, London.

Youle, A. (1995) The thermal environment. In: *Occupational Hygiene* (eds J.M. Harrington & K. Gardiner), pp. 191–226. Blackwell Science, Oxford.

4 Ventilation

Introduction

Where natural ventilation does not provide an adequate exchange of fresh air, mechanical devices such as fans may be provided to supply or extract air locally or to ventilate an environment in general. Where the air is required to be moved some distance, ducting is used that may be of considerable length and contain bends, changes of section, branch pieces and other fittings. Coupled with the capacity to draw in fresh air or to recirculate it, the system may contain filters, heaters, coolers, humidifiers or a combination of these and, to prevent atmospheric pollution from the discharge of dirty air, dust collectors and various air cleaners may be used. The performance of these ventilation systems needs to be checked from time to time to ensure their satisfactory operation. This may involve measuring air volume flow rates, velocities and pressures at extraction points and inside ducts. This can be supplemented by the tracing of air-flow patterns around ventilation terminals such as extraction hoods, slots, enclosures and fume cupboards. The routine checking of local exhaust ventilation is mandatory where it is used to control substances hazardous to health under the COSHH Regulations 1998 and where it is used to control airborne asbestos fibres under The Control of Asbestos at Work Regulations 1987. It is also desirable to check regularly the performance of ventilation systems that maintain a comfortable or a healthy working environment.

Natural ventilation is difficult to measure as it relies upon pressure differences created by natural forces such as the wind or differences in air temperature between inside and outside the building and therefore is constantly fluctuating unlike the more steady mechanically induced air flows. Nevertheless, natural air flows can be estimated using a technique outlined in this chapter. Air volume flow rates are quoted in units of cubic metres per second ($m^3 s^{-1}$) or in air changes per hour. For natural ventilation rates air changes per hour is more commonly used. This unit can be converted to $m^3 s^{-1}$ by multiplying it by the volume of the room in cubic metres and dividing the result by 3600. Air speeds are quoted in metres per second ($m s^{-1}$).

Air pressures are usually quoted as gauge pressures. That is, the pressure difference between inside the system and atmospheric pressure or that of the room in which the equipment is installed. In SI units pressure (p) is quoted in Newtons per square metre ($N m^{-2}$), which is also known as a Pascal (Pa), that is $1 Pa = 1 N m^{-2}$. However, as pressure gauges are often simple U-tubes containing a liquid such as water or paraffin, tradition has it that pressures are sometimes quoted as the length or height of a column of liquid, for example, inches or millimetres of water. In order to convert a column of liquid to Pascals the following equation is used:

$$p = \rho'gh \text{ Pa},$$

where ρ' = the density of the liquid in the guage in kg m^{-3}

h = the height of the column in metres, and

g = the acceleration due to gravity (9.81 m s^{-2})

Example: A column of water of height 100 mm expressed as a unit of pressure, Pa, is calculated knowing that the density of water is 1000 kg m^{-3} from

$$p = 1000 \times 9.81 \times \frac{100}{1000} = 981 \text{ Pa}$$

Some further explanation of pressure is necessary in order to differentiate between static pressure, velocity pressure and total pressure in ventilation systems.

Static pressure is the pressure exerted in all directions by a fluid that is stationary. If it is in motion it is the pressure exerted at right angles to the direction of flow. It can be either positive or negative. For example, on the suction side of a fan it would be negative but on the delivery side positive, in relation to atmospheric pressure.

Velocity pressure (p_v) is defined as the pressure equivalent of the kinetic energy of a fluid in motion but it is best illustrated as that pressure which is exerted on a surface placed across an airstream as in the sail of a boat or the vanes of a windmill thus causing them to move if sufficiently strong. It is calculated from the expression:

$$p_v = \rho \frac{v^2}{2} \text{ Pa}$$

Therefore $v = \sqrt{\dfrac{2p_v}{\rho}}$ or $\left(\dfrac{2p_v}{\rho}\right)^{\frac{1}{2}}$,

where ρ = the density of the air in kg m^{-3}, and

v = the velocity of the air in m s^{-1}

Velocity pressure is always positive.

Total pressure is the sum of the static and the velocity pressure at a point in an airstream and can be either positive or negative in relation to atmospheric pressure.

Equipment available

Pressure measuring instruments

It is possible to make a simple pressure gauge or 'manometer' by taking a glass tube bent in a U-shape and filling it half full with water. With one limb connected to the inside of the ventilation duct by means of rubber or plastic tubing at the point where the pressure is required, and with the other limb open to the atmosphere, the water will take up different levels in each limb. The difference in vertical height between the two liquid levels represents the pressure in the duct. Using the formula given above this pressure in Pascals can be calculated. For very low pressures this instrument will be imprecise because it will be difficult to measure the difference in height of the two columns. If more precision is required then it is necessary to incline one limb of the U-tube as in Fig. 4.1.

There is a range of commercially available manometers from simple vertical U-tubes to instruments whose angle of inclination can be varied in known fixed positions and whose scales are calibrated in various units of pressure. The liquids used in the more sophisticated instruments are usually of a lower specific gravity than water thus providing a more extended scale than with water for the same pressure. It is important to ensure that such gauges are

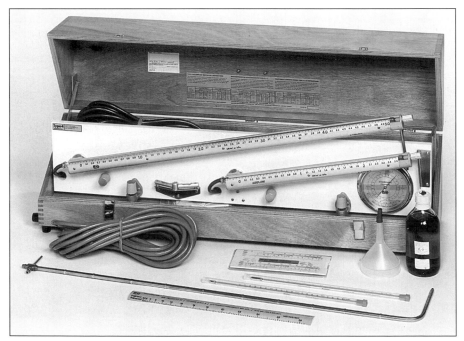

Fig. 4.1. Portable inclined manometer (Airflow Developments Ltd).

filled with the correct liquid or the scales will give the incorrect value. Also with gauges having variable inclinations it is important to multiply the reading obtained by a scale factor appropriate to the angle of inclination as provided by the manufacturer.

Liquid-filled gauges have the disadvantage that the liquid must be free of bubbles when being used. Over-loading the gauge can result in bubbles being formed or the liquid being blown out of the tubes. Also, vertical U-tubes must be held vertically when in use and inclined manometers must be carefully levelled and zeroed before use and kept level whilst being read.

Diaphragm gauges do not have these disadvantages as a reading is obtained on a dial by a pointer actuated by the movement of a diaphragm, one side of which is exposed to the pressure to be measured. A mechanical or magnetic linkage moves the pointer.

Such gauges are much easier to use in industrial situations but they need to be calibrated from time to time against an accurate inclined manometer set up under suitable laboratory conditions. They also require to be zeroed before taking a set of readings, which can be done by joining the two pressure tappings by a tube and making the appropriate adjustment. Gauges of this type can be read by placing either in a vertical or horizontal position but they must be zeroed in the plane in which they are to be used. An example of a diaphragm gauge is shown in Fig. 4.2.

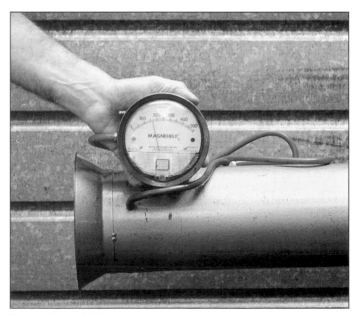

Fig. 4.2. Magnehelic diaphragm pressure gauge.

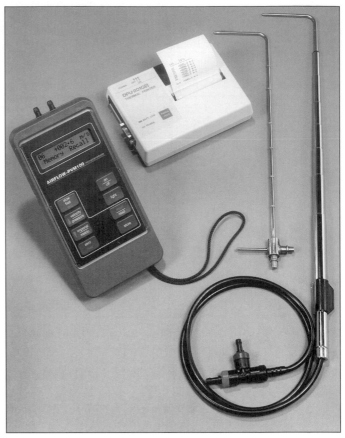

Fig. 4.3. Digital micromanometer (Airflow Developments Ltd).

A wide range of pressures can be measured using battery-powered micromanometers as illustrated in Figs 4.3 and 4.4. Displays can be digital or analogue and some have the facility to display an air velocity corresponding to a measured velocity pressure when coupled to a pitot-static tube (see pages 92–95), assuming standard air density.

Air velocity measuring instruments

There is a wide variety of air velocity instruments available and they can be classified into three main groups: vane anemometers, heated head anemometers and velocity pressure devices.

Vane anemometers

These are small rotating windmills mechanically or electrically coupled to a meter or a digital indicator. The mechanically coupled ones require to be used in conjunction with a timing device such as a stop-watch or electronic timer but the electrical vane anemometers

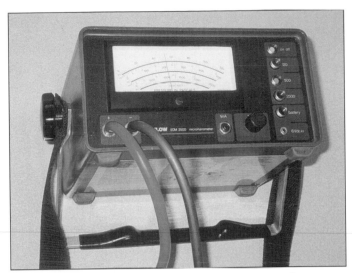

Fig. 4.4. Electronic micromanometer (Airflow Developments Ltd).

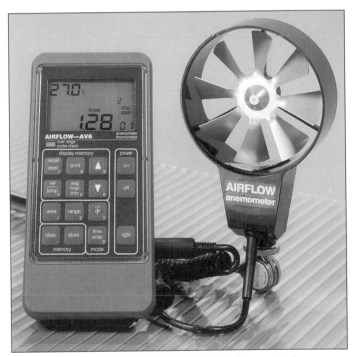

Fig. 4.5. Electrical vane anemometer (Airflow Developments Ltd).

(Fig. 4.5 and 4.6) give a direct reading in units of air velocity such as metres per second. The modern instruments are available in diameters varying from 100 mm to 25 mm but as the rotating vanes are extremely light and are suspended on jewelled bearings it is important to ensure that they are handled carefully and that nothing is allowed to touch the vanes. This type of instrument requires calibrating regularly if reliable results are to be obtained. The electrically powered instruments should not be used in flammable atmospheres unless they are certified intrinsically safe.

When using these instruments it must be borne in mind that they are sensitive to 'yaw', that is, their axis must be parallel to the airstream lines. The angle of yaw is the angle between the axis of the instrument and the airstream lines.

Heated head air meters

These devices rely upon the cooling power of the air to cool a sensitive head. Although the Kata thermometer mentioned in the chapter on heat measurement could be classified as one of these, it is not described here as it is only used to measure velocities of less than 0.5 m s^{-1}. Essentially the heated head is a hot wire, thermocouple or thermistor bead through which an electric current is passing to maintain it at a constant temperature. As air blows over it cooling takes place, the rate of cooling depending upon the air velocity. The current that is required to keep the temperature constant is registered on a meter, which has been previously calibrated in units of air velocity. An example of this is shown in Fig. 4.7. As with vane anemometers they require careful handling and regular calibration against known air speeds. Also they should not be used in flammable atmospheres.

Some of these instruments have a cowl over the sensing head to direct air over it which means that they must be carefully placed in the airstream with no yaw.

Velocity pressure devices

It is possible to measure velocity pressure using a pressure gauge as described above in conjunction with a probe known as a 'pitot-static' tube (Fig. 4.8). This device consists of two tubes, one concentrically placed inside the other. The inner tube is positioned facing into the airstream with its axis parallel to the stream lines sensing the total pressure. The outer tube is sealed at the end with an aerofoil-shaped seal allowing only a small opening for the inner tube. Around the outer tube is a ring of holes that are at right angles to the airstream sensing static pressure. At the opposite end to the sensing head the tubes are each fitted with a nozzle to connect to the pressure gauge via flexible tubing. In order to facilitate insertion into the side of ducting the whole device is bent at a right angle. The principle of operation is as follows: as the static pressure inside the duct is acting upon both tubes it is also acting upon each side of the pressure gauge and therefore cancels itself out leaving only the velocity pressure to provide the reading on the gauge. This is

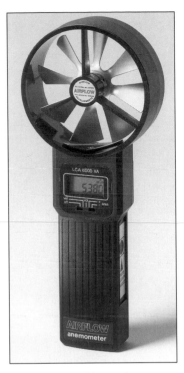

Fig. 4.6. Handheld averaging vane anemometer (Airflow Developments Ltd).

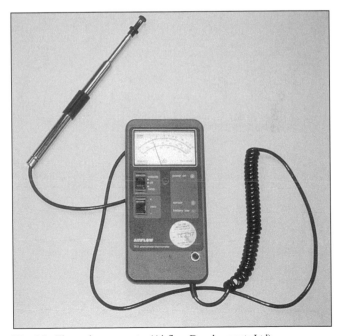

Fig. 4.7. Thermal anemometer (Airflow Developments Ltd).

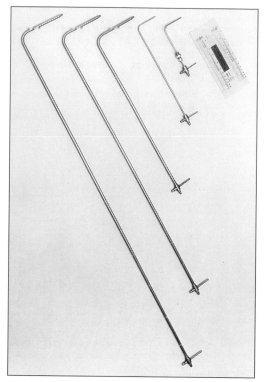

Fig. 4.8. Pitot-static tubes (Airflow Developments Ltd).

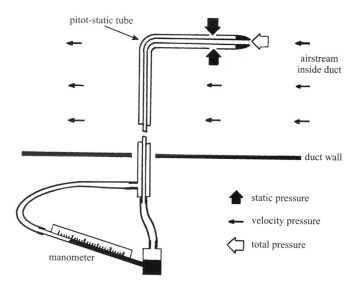

Fig. 4.9. Principle of operation of pitot-static tube.

illustrated diagramatically in Fig. 4.9. Rearranging the velocity pressure formula mentioned earlier the air velocity (v) can be calculated from the measured pressure as follows:

$$v = \sqrt{\frac{2\,p_v}{\rho}} \text{ m s}^{-1}$$

Example: a velocity pressure of 100 Pa is measured using a pitot-static tube, assuming air density is 1.2 kg m^{-3} the air velocity is:

$$v = \sqrt{\frac{2 \times 100}{1.2}} = 12.9 \text{ m s}^{-1}$$

It is important to note that this instrument is sensitive to air velocities above 3 m s^{-1} but below this precision is lost. If velocities are likely to be below 3 m s^{-1} an alternative air-flow meter should be used. Also, with pitot-static tubes, it is important to ensure that the tube points directly into the airstream since any deviation will result in errors. To this end some makes of pitot-static tube have a pointer at the lower end to indicate the direction in which the head is pointing. A pitot-static tube should only be used for duct velocities. It is unsuitable for measuring the velocity at the face of hoods or booths.

Smoke tube kit

To trace the patterns of air flow outside ducts, to spot leaks of air, to identify sources of draught, and to visualise turbulence, for example, at the edges of fume cupboards or booths, a smoke tracer is available. White smoke can be produced in a variety of ways but the most convenient one is to purchase a smoke tube kit, which consists of a rubber bulb fitted with one-way valves and a small sealed glass tube containing a chemical that, when exposed to air, gives off a stream of white smoke. To activate the chemical it is necessary to break the sealed ends of the glass tube and attach one end to the bulb. By squeezing the bulb air is passed through the tube producing a stream of white smoke. Rubber end seals can be fitted to the tube to conserve the chemical for later use. There is a tendency for the tube to seal itself with a deposit of white powder before all the chemical is exhausted but this can be cleared with a thin spike.

A useful feature of smoke produced this way is that it is at the same temperature as the surrounding air. It is not recommended that cigarette smoke be used as it is hotter than the surrounding air and will tend to rise, giving a false picture of the air-flow patterns.

Sometimes it is necessary to use larger clouds of smoke than can be produced from a tube kit. For example, to trace the stack of a chemical fume cupboard amongst many in a laboratory block or to observe the behaviour of a plume leaving the stack. Larger, more stable and continuous streams of smoke can be produced using an ignitable chemical smoke producer similar to fireworks and supplied by firework manufacturers. A theatrical smoke machine is also useful; this relies on large quantities of white fumes produced when glycerol is dropped on a hotplate, which is blown out by a fan integral to the machine. This device is a standard method of visually testing the containment of a chemical fume cupboard in some countries.

Calibration devices

It is necessary to check the performance of air velocity instruments from time to time against accurately known air speeds. This is best done in a wind tunnel but such devices are large, expensive and are limited in location to the larger research establishments and universities, and may not be easily accessible. However, there is a small, relatively inexpensive wind tunnel commercially available known as an 'open jet' wind tunnel, which can guarantee air velocities to within ± 2% of the true value. This is sufficiently precise for most field measurements. The device can be installed on an open bench provided there is at least 6 m of unrestricted horizontal space available. A description of the method of use of this tunnel is given later.

Barometric pressure instruments

Barometric pressure can be measured by a variety of devices. The absolute instrument is the Fortin barometer, which is a column of mercury contained in an inverted sealed tube standing in a trough of mercury. The column is held up by air pressure whose value is expressed by the height of the column supported in millimetres. For example, standard atmospheric pressure is 760 mm of mercury (Hg). This value can be converted into Pascal and hence into bar or millibar (mb) by using the formula on page 87 (1 bar = 10^5 Pa or 1 mb = 100 Pa). This pressure is also measured by an aneroid barometer, which is essentially a sealed bellows-type chamber that expands and contracts with changes in pressure and moves a needle on a suitably calibrated dial. The latest devices use pressure transducers, which can provide a signal to a digital display.

Ventilation measurement records

In accordance with Regulation 9 of the COSHH Regulations and the associated Code of Practice, statutory measurements and records of those measurements are required to be kept for at least 5 years. For routine measurements to be of any value the current performance figures need to be compared with the previous ones to obtain a trend. In this way the capability of the system to control can be judged.

In order to provide records, typical pro-formas are given in the Appendix to this chapter. The first two forms constitute a statement of the design specification of the ventilation system and includes a space for a sketch or photograph of its layout. The last two show the results of the regular routine measurements and could be used as often as required. For example, the COSHH Regulations require measurements to be made at intervals not greater than 14 months, but for many systems more frequent examination and monitoring may be required.

If the system is used to control large quantities of hazardous materials then the performance of the system may deteriorate due to heavy deposits on certain parts such as dampers and fan blades. On the other hand, the substance may react with the materials making up the control system and damage them. For example, acid vapour mists could corrode the ducting if made of certain metals. This emphasises the importance of including health and safety professionals at the design stage of the control system so that appropriate systems are selected and installed. Regulation 9 was written specifically to highlight and overcome problems of this sort.

The measurement of air flow in ducts

Aim
Ducted ventilation systems require checking at regular intervals to ensure that the designed air-flow rate is being maintained. Deterioration occurs gradually due to a variety of factors, but mainly because of a build-up of deposits on the fan blades, duct walls and other parts of the system. If a record of the results is routinely made, then trends can be spotted and remedial action taken.

Equipment required
An air speed measuring device – which can be either a vane anemometer, a heated head air velocity meter or a pitot-static tube and pressure gauge – a tape measure and a marker pen are needed. It should be borne in mind that whatever instrument is chosen, an access hole or holes are required in the duct wall to allow the instrument to be inserted, thus the smaller the instrument the smaller the hole. In this respect, the pitot-static tube is the most suitable, requiring a hole no larger than about 12 mm in diameter, although some of the smaller heated head instruments will also fit that size hole. Vane anemometers are less suitable for this purpose.

Note that if the ducting handles air containing radioactive, pathogenic material or toxic chemicals, then drilling holes may lead to contamination of the drill, the measuring instruments and escape of the pollutant into an occupied area.

Method

1 Select a suitable length of duct in the airstream to be measured. Ideally the measuring station should be in an airstream free from turbulence, which means the ducting should be straight and there should be no obstruction or changes of direction in the duct for at least 10 diameters upstream of it and none should appear downstream for 5 diameters. In many installations it is not possible to find such a place, therefore the longest length of straight ducting should be chosen and the measuring station taken as far downstream as possible from the last cause of turbulence. Unfortunately, the reliability of the results will be affected by the degree of turbulence in the airstream.

2 Having chosen a measuring station it is necessary to place the instrument's sensing head in representative places over the cross-section of the duct in order to obtain an average velocity. This is because the air moves at a higher speed towards the centre than it does close to the walls of the duct. The British Standard BS 848 recommends positions for the instrument as set out in Figs 4.10 and 4.11 for circular and rectangular cross-sections. Circular ducts are divided according to a log–linear rule and the rectangular according to a log Tchebycheff rule. Thus it may be necessary to drill various holes in the duct walls to suit the size of the measuring station. Plugs of rubber or other suitable material should be available to cover the holes after use.

3 In order to assist in placing the sensing head of the instrument in the correct position inside the duct, the stem or carrying arm should be marked so that when the mark is aligned with the side of the duct the head is in one of the positions indicated by Figs 4.10 or 4.11. For example, if the duct is circular in cross-section and of 300 mm diameter, the stem should be marked at the following six distances from the head:

$300 \times 0.032 = 9.6$ mm $\qquad$ $300 \times 0.679 = 203.7$ mm

$300 \times 0.135 = 40.5$ mm $\qquad$ $300 \times 0.865 = 259.5$ mm

$300 \times 0.321 = 96.3$ mm $\qquad$ $300 \times 0.968 = 290.4$ mm

Note: with some pitot-static tubes the stem has rings of spring steel, that can be adjusted to mark the appropriate position.

4 With battery-driven instruments, check the battery as indicated by the maker and turn on the meter and, where necessary, zero the scale in still air. This can be done by placing the head in a small closed container such as a tube sealed at one end.

5 With pitot-static tubes it is necessary to set up the pressure gauge. Inclined manometers require to be levelled and zeroed, but this is best done after the connecting tubes have been attached so as not to disturb the setting by so doing. The high-pressure side of

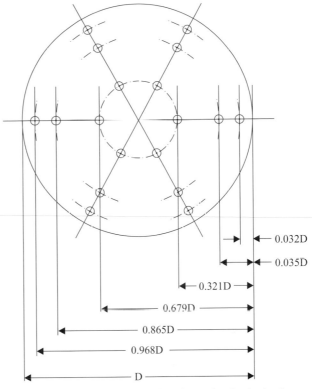

Fig. 4.10. Measuring positions for placing pitot-static tubes in circular ducting. Based on BS848 Part 1 (British Standards Institution, 1980).

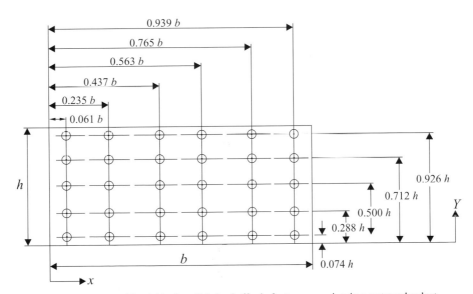

Fig. 4.11. Log Tchebycheff rule for traverse points in a rectangular duct. Based on BS848 Part 1 (British Standards Institution, 1980).

the gauge must be connected to the central tube of the pitot-static tube and the low-pressure side to the outside tube. Diaphragm gauges must be zeroed in the position in which they are to be read, i.e. either flat or vertical, but the position must not be changed after that.

6 Remove any protective cover from the sensing head and insert it through the hole in the duct and position it so that the first mark is against the duct wall. If the duct is circular, then the stem of the instrument must be held along the line of the diameter, but if it is a rectangular cross-section then the stem must be at right angles to the duct wall. Ensure that the sensing head is exactly facing into the airstream. This is important with instruments that have a directional shield around the head and with pitot-static tubes, which often have a pointer at the lower end to indicate the position in which the head is facing. Some heated head instruments have no directional characteristics so this is not important. When using pitot-static tubes and liquid filled manometers it is a wise precaution to bend and squeeze both flexible connecting tubes to cut off the pressure in the gauge, releasing them simultaneously only when the pitot-static tube is in the correct position. Alternatively, use a simultaneous switching device available with some liquid filled manometers. This can prevent an excessively high static pressure from blowing the fluid out of the gauge. If the air temperature and barometric pressure are very different from standard conditions (20 °C and 1013 mb), then they should also be measured.

7 Note the reading of the meter or the gauge and convert it to Pascals according to the scale factor or the conversion factor.

8 Move the head to the next position and repeat 7 and so on until all positions in the diagram have been measured.

9 It is wise to repeat the complete set of readings at least once more.

10 Where necessary measure duct temperature and obtain barometric pressure close to the measuring station.

11 Obtain the internal dimensions of the measuring station either by direct measurement, manufacturer's data or, in the case of a thick-walled duct, by measuring the outside dimensions and subtracting the thickness of the walls.

Calculation

Where air velocity meters have been used, it is necessary to correct each reading from the latest calibration chart for the instrument concerned. The corrected velocities in each set of results should then be averaged to obtain the average air velocity at the measuring station.

The pitot-static tube and gauge method has obtained a set of velocity pressure readings, which must be converted to a velocity before calculating an average. *Do not average the pressure readings.*

Calculate the air velocity as follows:

$$v = \sqrt{\frac{2 p_v}{\rho}} \text{ m s}^{-1}$$

where

p_v = the reading of the velocity pressure in Pa, and

ρ = the air density in kg m^{-3} which can be taken as 1.2 kg m^{-3}, unless the air temperature or barometric pressure is very different from 20 °C of 1013 mb which are standard conditions.

To correct for temperature and pressure:

$$\text{new density } \rho_1 = \frac{1.2 \times P_{at} \times 293}{1013 \times (273 + t)} \text{ kg m}^{-3}$$

Use ρ_1 in place of ρ in the above formula, where

P_{at} = barometric pressure in millibars (mb)

t = duct air temperature in °C

The volume of air flowing (Q) is calculated from the formula:

$$Q = \bar{v} A \text{ m}^3 \text{ s}^{-1}$$

where $\bar{v}$ = the average air velocity at the measuring station in m s^{-1}, that is, the arithmetic mean of the velocities measured at that measuring station, which could be the mean of 30 readings in a rectangular duct, or 20 or 24 in a circular duct, and

A = the cross-sectional area of the duct at the measuring station in m^2.

With circular cross-section:

$$A = \frac{\pi d^2}{4} \text{ m}^2$$

where d = diameter of duct in metres;
and with rectangular cross-section

$$A = a \times b \text{ m}^2$$

where a and b are the dimensions of the two sides of the rectangular duct at the measuring station.

Example: In order to measure the volume flow rate in a circular cross-section duct whose diameter was 200 mm, a six-point traverse was undertaken using a pitot-static tube and manometer. The following velocity pressures were obtained:

210, 213, 224, 230, 219, 214 (Pa).

Air temperature in the duct was 25 °C and the barometric pressure was measured to be 982 mb, which are non-standard conditions. Calculation of volume flow rate:

To calculate the new non-standard air density:

$$\rho = \frac{1.2 \times 293 \times b}{1013 \ (273+t)} \ \text{kg m}^{-3}$$

$$= 1.2 \times \frac{982 \times (273+20)}{1013 \ (273+25)} \ \text{kg m}^{-3}$$

$$= 1.14 \ \text{kg m}^{-3}$$

$$v = \sqrt{\frac{2 \, p_v}{\rho}} \ \text{m s}^{-1}$$

v (at each traverse point): $v_1 = \sqrt{\dfrac{2 \times 210}{1.14}} = 19.2 \text{ms}^{-1}$

$$v_2 = \sqrt{\frac{2 \times 213}{1.14}} = 19.3 \text{ms}^{-1}$$

Similarly $v_3 = 19.8 \text{ ms}^{-1}$

$$v_4 = 20.1 \text{ ms}^{-1}$$

$$v_5 = 19.6 \text{ ms}^{-1}$$

$$v_6 = 19.4 \text{ ms}^{-1}$$

$$\bar{v} = \frac{19.2 + 19.3 + 19.8 + 20.1 + 19.6 + 19.4}{6}$$

$$= 19.6 \text{ m s}^{-1}$$

$$A \ (\text{dia. } 0.2 \text{m}) = \frac{(0.2)^2 \pi}{4}$$

$$= 0.031 \text{m}^2$$

$$Q = vA \ \text{m}^3 \text{s}^{-1}$$

$$= 19.6 \times 0.031$$

$$= 0.62 \ \text{m}^3 \text{s}^{-1}$$

Note: the calculations are only to three significant figures as the precision of ventilation measurements of this nature is unlikely to be greater that ± 2%.

Possible problems

1   Ventilation flow rates fluctuate for a variety of reasons:
   (a)   some fans have a fluctuating output;
   (b)   external influences such as wind and weather can affect flow rates; and
   (c)   internal influences such as the movement of large loads across the entrance or exit of a ventilation system can affect flow rates. Therefore, it is important to take more than one set of readings.

2   Some flow rates pulsate, so, when reading meters, some estimate of the mid-point of the pulse should be taken.

3   Due to deposits of dust or sticky particles on the insides of ducting, the cross-sectional area may not be as expected. This is particularly prevalent in the ducting on paint spray booths. Adjustments can only be made by inspection.

The measurement of pressure in ventilation systems

Aim

In order that air should flow in ventilation systems it is necessary to create a pressure difference between the inside of the duct and the atmosphere. This is usually achieved by means of a fan. If the ducting is connected to the suction side of the fan the pressure inside is negative, thus drawing air into the system. A positive pressure is found on the discharge side, thus ducting on that side will deliver air under the influence of that pressure. Pressure is absorbed by the ducting, fittings and obstructions such as dampers and filters. With some ventilation systems dirt can build up inside, which can restrict the flow and increase the pressure absorbed. Also, fabric filters will gradually increase in resistance as dust is collected, resulting in an increase in pressure absorbed. It is, therefore, useful to measure pressures at various places in the system and, if done routinely, the trend can provide an indication of any deterioration in performance.

Equipment required

A manometer or diaphragm gauge, flexible plastic tubing of sufficient length to suit the siting of the gauge in relation to the measuring point (if pressure is to be measured on either side of an item, then it is useful to have tubing of two different colours), some moulding clay or plasticine to act as a sealant, a hand or electric drill capable of drilling holes the same diameter as the outside diameter of the flexible tubing, some rubber plugs or tape to seal up the hole after measuring.

Method

1   Select places to insert the tubing to suit the requirements of the system. For example, on either side of a filter, on either side of the fan, and/or at chosen places along the ducting. Drill a hole into the duct at each place. If the site is to be measured regularly then it may be advantageous and labour saving if a permanent nozzle is soldered or fixed to the duct wall at the hole to take the flexible tubing. The inner edge of the nozzle must be flush with the inside of the duct so that none protrudes into the airstream, and a cap should be fitted to prevent leakage after use.

Note: that if the ducting handles air containing radioactive, pathogenic material or toxic chemicals, then drilling holes may lead to contamination of the drill, the measuring instruments and escape of the pollutant into an occupied area.

2   Connect a length of flexible plastic tubing to each side of the gauge.

3   Level and zero the gauge.

4   Using the highest pressure range available, connect the other ends of the tubing to the places to be measured. With liquid filled manometers it is necessary to think carefully about the pressures to be measured before connecting the tubing into the system, as liquid can easily be removed by the ventilation pressure. The following points should be borne in mind:

    (a)   positive pressure will depress and negative pressure elevate the liquid in the limb to which it is connected;

    (b)   if a gauge pressure is to be measured, that is, with one side of the gauge open to atmosphere, then all parts of the ventilation system on the suction side of the fan will be at a negative pressure, whilst those on the delivery side will be at a positive pressure;

    (c)   if a pressure difference is to be measured between two parts of the system – that is, both tubes are connected into the ducting – then, with the exception of the fans themselves, the air flows from the high to the low pressure, which means that the upstream side will be at the higher pressure;

    (d)   with fans the higher pressure will be on the delivery side.

5   Having selected the highest range, if the pressure reading is low then a lower range can be used.

6   Note the reading, remove the tubing and seal the hole.

7   The recorded value must be multiplied by the scale factor of the range used.

Results

Little information can be gained from the results unless the design values of the system are known, against which the measurements can be compared. However, if routine measurements are taken, say once every month, and a continuous record kept then the condition of the ventilation system can be observed regularly, and if any deterioration is noted then corrective action can be taken. It is suggested that for each measuring station a record sheet be kept containing the information, as shown in the Appendix at the end of this chapter.

Possible problems

1   Ventilation pressures may fluctuate due to external influences. If this is the case, then the cause should be removed if possible and the readings repeated.

2   If the pressure continues to fluctuate or pulsate then a mean or mid-point of the pulsation must be taken.

3   If the ventilation pressure has been misjudged when using a liquid filled gauge and the liquid has bubbled or blown out, then it is important to ensure that the flexible tubing is cleared of fluid and the liquid replenished in the gauge and all bubbles removed. It may be necessary to hang the tubing in a vertical position to drain for some time or to blow it through with a jet of compressed air. Bubbles may be removed by gently rocking the fluid in the gauge from side to side using a blowing action through a short length of clean tubing.

To measure the face velocity on a booth or hood

Aim

Fume cupboards, paint spray booths and other ventilated enclosures control the emission of substances by providing an enclosure on five of the six sides around the source, and on the sixth maintaining an inward velocity of air such that the pollutants released in the enclosure could not escape. The velocity maintained on the open face is known as the 'face velocity' and for most situations should be kept within the range $0.5-2.5$ m s^{-1}. The aperture height could be critical when highly toxic materials are handled. An indication of the average velocity plus a profile of the range of velocities at different points across the face is required.

Equipment required

A rotating vane anemometer or heated head instrument, tape measure and marker pen. Some rotating vane anemometers have the facility to provide an average velocity over a period of time determined by the measurer. Such an instrument would be useful in this instance.

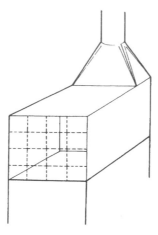

Fig. 4.12. Face of booth showing measuring positions.

Method

Using a tape measure and marker pen, the face of the enclosure should be divided into imaginary rectangles as shown in Fig. 4.12. The air velocity measuring instrument should be held in the centre of the imaginary rectangle and allowed to remain there for a few seconds to adjust to a steady speed (the larger the diameter of the vane anemometer the longer it will take to reach this speed). The reading should be noted on a sketch of the face with the positions and distances labelled. When noted, move to the next rectangle and so on until the whole face is measured.

It is advisable to repeat all readings at least three times or until consistent readings are obtained.

Results

Using the calibration chart of the air speed instrument used, correct all the readings taken to provide the true velocity. Examine the individual spot readings to ascertain if any parts of the face have an inconsistent reading, such as too low or too high, and try to establish the reason. A velocity below 0.5 m s^{-1} at any one spot may result in pollutants escaping into the breathing zone of the worker from that position. It is useful to make an arithmetic mean of the face veolcities, then check each reading to see whether it is in within ± 20% of that mean. If any is, then the reason should be sought and the condition remedied. If the velocity profile looks reasonably even, calculate the arithmetic mean of the spot readings to present as the average face velocity and note it.

Possible problems

1   With a hand-held instrument it is possible to affect the readings by having an arm or other part of the body too close to the face, thus creating air currents that are not typical of normal conditions. Care should be taken to ensure that the minimum of obstruction is caused by the measurer and the instrument.

2   If the velocity profile is very uneven such that at some places the velocity is virtually zero, that is, the vane anemometer ceases to rotate, then an unsatisfactory situation is indicated, which should be noted and rectified as soon as possible. Furthermore, the average velocities obtained would be imprecise and of little value.

To measure the face velocity on a chemical fume cupboard

Aim

Chemical fume cupboards are a special type of enclosure having a sliding front cover or sash. This serves two purposes: it protects the eyes and face of the operator from splashing of chemicals released inside, and it improves the enclosure by partially enclosing the sixth side, i.e. the front. The position of the sash may affect the velocity of the entering air as the area of opening will vary. The aim is to ensure that the face velocity is within a range dictated by the degree of hazard being contained, as follows:

Situation	Recommended face velocity m s^{-1}
Low toxicity substances	0.4
General use	0.5
Radiotoxic and highly toxic substances	0.75
For spraying chromatograms	0.9

Any measurements taken should be combined with inspections of the condition of the structure and services provided in the fume cupboard and the free movement of the sash. All defects should be reported.

Equipment required

A rotating vane or heated head anemometer, tape measure and marker pen. Some rotating vane anemometers have the facility to provide an average velocity over a period of time or over a series of measuring positions. Such an instrument may be useful for this exercise.

Method

Set the sash to the normal operating position. In well-regulated laboratories this will normally be indicated by an arrow on the side of the frame.

Using the tape measure and marker pen divide the face into imaginary rectangles similar to those shown in Fig. 4.12. As a general guide, the rectangles should have the long side between 200–300 mm and the short side between 100–200 mm, depending upon the area of opening.

Hold the air velocity meter in the centre of each marked rectangle and allow it to remain there for a few seconds before noting the reading. Write down the results on a sketch of the face with the positions and dimensions labelled.

Having noted the reading, move to the next rectangle and repeat until all the rectangles have been measured.

Results

Using the calibration chart of the air velocity instrument correct all readings to obtain the true velocities.

Make an arithmetic mean of the face velocities and check against the recommended face velocity. If the mean is below the recommended it may be necessary to close the sash to achieve the correct value. In this case, the arrow marking the normal operating position must be moved to indicate the new sash position. Also, check each reading to see whether it is within ± 20% of that mean. If any is, then the reason should be sought and the condition remedied.

Possible problems

The position of equipment inside the fume cupboard may influence individual readings. This is particularly so if it is too close to the front. Ask the operator whether the equipment can be placed further inside the cupboard and if possible move it. Not only will this improve the distribution of velocities on the face it will probably reduce any risk of pollutants escaping.

Note: most fume cupboards have a device to ensure a reasonably constant face velocity whatever the position of the sash and to prevent excessively high velocities when the sash is nearly fully closed. This may take the form of a by-pass grille or duct or by means of a variable speed fan. Do not estimate the volume flow rate of the fan by using the face velocity unless the sash is in the fully opened position as some air may be flowing through the by-pass.

Face velocity measurements may be combined with fan inlet flow rate and static pressure and, where possible, discharge stack velocity.

To measure the performance of a suction inlet

Aim
Extract hoods, slots, enclosures and fume cupboards are intended to capture air pollutants to prevent them from being released into the general room atmosphere. Unfortunately many have insufficient air flowing or have their suction inlet too far away from the point of release of the pollutant, or they have inadequate enclosure around the source. Thus, some means of checking the air-flow patterns and air velocity in and around the inlet is useful so that the full extent of the zone of influence of the device can be ascertained.

Equipment required
A smoke tube kit, a tape measure and an air speed indicator such as a thermistor bead flowmeter or a vane anemometer (the former is to be preferred as it will record at lower air speeds and is less sensitive to air direction) are needed. Ideally a thermistor bead instrument with an unshielded head would be best.

Method
It should be pointed out at this stage that this method is intended to trace air flow patterns and measure air velocities around the inlet and not to check on the absolute efficiency of the suction device. To achieve the latter it would be necessary to release a tracer gas whose decay of airborne concentration with distance from the source could be measured using some direct reading analysis instrument.

1   Ensure that cross-draughts and local air turbulence is minimised during the test. For example, close doors or windows and restrict the movement of people in the vicinity. In particularly busy workplaces it may be necessary to undertake this work outside working hours.

2   Break the ends of the smoke tube and insert it in the rubber bulb, puff smoke around the suction inlet gradually moving further away from the mouth until the full extent of the zone of influence can be observed. The places where the smoke is no longer being drawn in marks the edge of the zone of influence of this inlet.

3   Make a sketch drawing of the inlet and the equipment of the workplace that lies within the zone of influence.

4   Plot on the sketch an imaginary grid of squares across the face of the inlet and in the area in front to cover the whole zone of influence in the horizontal plane containing the source of pollutant. Other planes, both vertical and horizontal, can be chosen if a full picture is required. The dimensions of the grid squares should be 100–150 mm depending upon the size of the inlet, the smaller ones using the smaller squares.

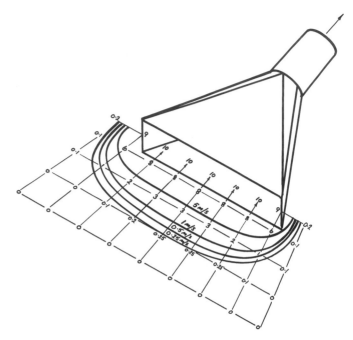

Fig. 4.13. Extract slot showing a horizontal grid on the centre line with measured air velocity results and plotted contours.

5   Using the tape measure as a guide to the measuring positions place the sensing head at the corner of each grid square taking care to ensure that the instrument is, as far as possible, axial to the airstreams' lines. This may be difficult as the airstreams around suction inlets are curved as air enters from all sides. Also the sensing head should be carried on a long probe so that the position of the observer's arms and body does not interfere with the flow patterns. Note the air velocity at each place by writing it on the sketch at the appropriate position (Fig. 4.13).

6   Measure the air velocity on the face of the inlet along the centre line at the intersection with each of the grid lines. Note the results on the sketch. If there is a flat surface in front of the hood, such as a work bench, do not allow the instrument head to touch the surface but lift it clear of the surface, level with the centreline of the hood.

7   Repeat item 5 above for as many planes as have been chosen.

Results

Correct each reading using the appropriate calibration chart. Make an average of the velocities across the face of the inlet and note the range of the readings in relation to the average. If there is a wide variation then the air flow distribution is uneven and may require some means of equalisation using face slots or air flow splitters or guides.

Inspect the results on any chosen plane of grids and try to estimate the position of points of equal velocity. For example, draw a cross or spot at the points, where in your opinion, the 10, 5, 1, 0.5 and 0.25 m s^{-1} velocities occur. Join up the spots of equal velocity to produce a velocity contour of that air speed as shown in Fig. 4.13. The lowest contour should be 0.25 m s^{-1}. Any pollutant released outside this contour is unlikely to be captured or drawn into the inlet even if released into an undisturbed airstream, and if turbulence is caused by cross-draughts due to the presence of external influences such as open windows, doors or the movement of people or vehicles then pollutant will escape the zone of influence and be released into the general air.

The measurement of natural air infiltration rate in a room

Aim

It is normally possible to obtain an indication of the air-flow rate in a room that is mechanically ventilated, as the majority of the air flowing will pass through the fan or duct serving the room, but with rooms that rely on infiltration of air by seepage through the building fabric and around doors and windows it is much more difficult. It may be important to know the flow rate in order to calculate heat losses or to establish whether a room requires to be mechanically ventilated for a particular purpose, or it may be useful to know just how 'leaky' the room is. The impracticability of trying to measure flow rates around doors and windows and cracks in the building fabric is obvious; thus, an alternative technique must be used. With most rooms the natural infiltration rate will depend upon external influences, particularly the wind; therefore, any result obtained must be related to wind speed and direction. An exercise such as this must be repeated several times over a variety of weather conditions in order to obtain a fair assessment of the natural flow rates, since one single measurement is virtually meaningless.

Equipment required

A supply of tracer gas such as nitrous oxide, sulphur hexafluoride or radioactive krypton (^{85}Kr), a detector capable of measuring concentrations of the chosen gas at low levels, a desk fan, a timer, a sheet of log-linear graph paper and an anemometer.

Method

The method described here uses the tracer gas ^{85}Kr and a Geiger–Muller tube and counter as the detector, but the procedure is essentially the same regardless of the tracer gas and detector used. The principle involved is to release a quantity of the tracer gas into the room and to measure how quickly it is diluted by the infiltration air.

1   Adjust the room to the conditions for which the measurements are needed, that is, shut the doors and windows or leave certain of them open as required.

2   Place the desk fan and Geiger–Muller tube on a table in the centre of the room and pass the cables out under the door. Connect the Geiger cable to the counter situated outside the room in the corridor or adjacent room and measure the background count.

3   Start the desk fan, which should be switched from outside the room.

4   Enter the room and break an ampoule of 74 MBq (2 mCi) of ^{85}Kr on a tray provided to capture the broken glass and leave the room immediately.

5   Wait for 5 minutes to allow the desk fan and diffusion forces to mix the gas thoroughly with the air in the room.

6   Switch off the fan and measure the number of counts per minute from the Geiger counter. Continue to note the counts per minute at 5-minute intervals until the concentration of the gas has been diluted to a level approaching the measured background or for 45 minutes, whichever is the shorter. (In the case of a tracer gas other than ^{85}Kr being used, note the concentration as measured by the detector every 5 minutes over a 45-minute period.)

7   Re-enter the room and open all windows to clear the remaining gas.

8   Measure the wind speed and direction at a place that represents the true effect on the building, such as the roof or at an open space adjacent.

Calculations

The air-flow rate in number of air changes per hour is calculated from the expression:

$$N = \frac{1}{t}\left[\log_e C_o - \log_e C_t\right]$$

where N = the number of air changes per hour

t = the time between chosen concentrations in hours

C_o = the first concentration

C_t = the concentration after time t.

Subtract the background count from all readings and choose two readings, one from the start of the test and one near the end, and substitute in the above expression using t as the time interval between the two readings. Note that most scientific electronic calculators have a $\log_e$ or 1n function, which will simplify this calculation.

Example:

Background count = 40.

Readings taken:

Time (min)	Count (per min)	Corrected count (per min)
0	1520	1480
+5	861	821
+10	300	260
+15	256	216
+20	170	130
+25	105	65
+30	75	35
+35	65	25
+40	56	16

Taking counts at time = 0 and time = + 35 min, C_o = 1480, C_t = 25, t = 35/60 hours.

Air change rate N = 60/35 [$\log_e 1480 - \log_e 25$] = 7 air changes per hour. An alternative graphical solution can be made by plotting on log-linear graph paper, the corrected count (or gas concentration) on the log scale against time on the linear scale and drawing a straight line through the points. The slope of this curve represents the number of air changes per hour.

To convert air changes per hour to $m^3 \, s^{-1}$ multiply by the volume of the room in cubic metres and divide by 3600.

Calibration of an anemometer in an open jet wind tunnel

Aim

To check the accuracy of an air-flow measuring device and to provide a calibration chart for the range of the instrument.

Equipment required

An open jet wind tunnel as shown in Fig. 4.14, orifice plates, manometer (inclined gauge), dry bulb thermometer, anemometer stand as supplied with the tunnel or a retort stand, a barometer.

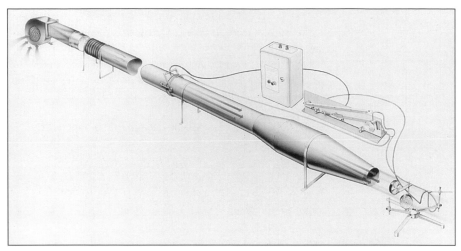

Fig. 4.14. Open jet wind tunnel (Airflow Developments Ltd).

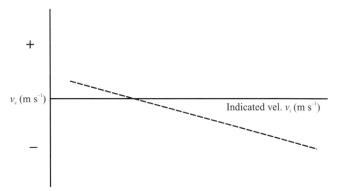

Fig. 4.15. Typical calibration chart for anemometer.

Method

1 Read and record tunnel air temperature in degrees Centigrade and room barometric pressure in millimetres of mercury.

2 Mount the anemometer to be tested 150 mm from the discharge nozzle. Make sure that the direction of flow through the instrument is correct and that the face of the instrument is at right angles to the air jet and placed centrally. A template should be made to ensure this.

3 Select and mount an orifice plate for the velocity range to be tested.

4 Set up and zero the manometer and connect it by means of flexible plastic tubing to the pressure tappings on each side of the orifice plate, the high pressure side being the nearest to the fan.

5 Switch on the fan and by means of the controlling rheostat adjust the air flow rate so that the anemometer dial reads a whole number.

6   Record the anemometer indicated flow rate and the orifice plate pressure difference as indicated on the manometer. Multiply this pressure reading by the appropriate scale factor for the angle of inclination of the gauge.

7   Alter the air flow rate and repeat until four results are obtained from the orifice plate.

8   Change the orifice plate and repeat so that four results are obtained from each orifice plate.

9   Record all results taken on a table similar to that shown in the Appendix to this chapter.

Results and calculations

Calculate air density correction factor (d) from:

$$d = \sqrt{\left(\frac{760}{b} \times \frac{273+t}{293}\right)}$$

where t = tunnel air temperature in °C, and

   b = barometric pressure in mmHg.

Calculate the 'true air velocity' (v_a) for each pressure reading from:

$$v_a = Ad\sqrt{\Delta p} \text{ m s}^{-1}$$

where Δp = the orifice plate differential pressure Pa, and

   A = calibration constant for each orifice plate.

Calculate the corrected velocity (v_c) for each reading from:

$$v_c = v_a - v_i$$

Plot v_c against v_i on a graph whose ordinates are shown in Fig. 4.15.

To complete a ventilation record

When checking the performance of extract ventilation systems it is necessary to have a record of the details of the system against which to compare the routine measurements. The following information should be available:

Identification details – the name and number of the plant; its location; the type of plant; the hazardous substances that are being controlled.

Enclosures and hoods – maximum number to be in use at any time; location or position; static pressure behind each hood or extraction point; face velocity.

Ducting – dimensions; transport velocity; volume flow.

Filter/collector – specification; volume flow; static pressure at inlet, outlet and across filter.

Fan or air mover – specification; volume flow; static pressure at inlet; direction and speed of rotation.

Systems that return exhaust air to the workplace – filter efficiency; concentration of contamination in return air. The majority of items on this list are taken from paragraph 66 of the Approved Code of Practice of the United Kingdom COSHH Regulations 1994. Whether this information is required by law or not, the more that is known about the ventilation system the easier it is to understand what it is trying to do. If changes are required then it is easier to make a decision as to the capacity of the system to cope with the new proposals.

A proforma on which to record this information is given on pages 1 and 2 of the Appendix to this chapter. However, unless the system is new and the design specification known some of it may be difficult to obtain and some guidance is given below.

Identification details – the first part of page 1 identifies the company, the plant items with the company's reference number, the department and the location. The hazardous substance or substances controlled by the plant should be identified, together with the published occupational exposure limits for those substances. These are obtained from the latest copy of the statutory standards for the country of application. For example, in the UK the latest HSE Publication EH40/– should be consulted. It is also useful to describe the ventilation system, for example a typical entry might be as follows: 'a multi-branched extract drawing air from four welding booths through flexible arm hoods', or 'a chemical fume cupboard fitted with a single fan discharging to atmosphere'. The description need not be too detailed as the sketch in page 2 will provide more information.

Below this introductory information the form examines each of the plant items, such as the fan, the filters, or the suction inlets (hoods etc.). The ductwork can be described in the sketch with the duct dimension written by each length. The dimensions of the ducts leading from the hoods etc. can be inserted in the extract points section of the table.

The fan specification – this section will identify the fan maker and the serial number. This is usually found on a plate riveted to the fan casing. In some instances this is missing or the plate is so corroded

Table 4.1. Results sheet for open jet wind tunnel calibration test

Orifice plate	Diameter (mm)	Calibration constant A*	Recommended velocity/range (m s^{-1})	Indicated velocity v_i (m s^{-1})	Orifice plate pressure differential Δp (Pa)	True air velocity v_a (m s^{-1})	Velocity correction v_c (m s^{-1})
1	33.2	0.0325	0.2–0.9	1	1		
				2	2		
				3	3		
				4	4		
2	72.2	0.174	0.75–5.0	1	1		
				2	2		
				3	3		
				4	4		
3	101.6	0.356	2.5–10.0	1	1		
				2	2		
				3	3		
				4	4		
4	163.8	1.168	5.0–30.0	1	1		
				2	2		
				3	3		
				4	4		

* This constant is specific to an individual wind tunnel and orifice plate and should be supplied by the manufacturer or obtained by calibration.

that it cannot be read, in which case 'information not available' should be entered. The type of fan is usually obvious by inspection. The most common fans are either axial flow or centrifugal, the former normally being cylindrical in shape with a propeller type of impeller rotating inside and an electrical cable attached to a junction box on the casing. The centrifugal fan has a casing that is scroll-shaped with the inlet duct entering at the centre and the outlet duct connected to the periphery, i.e. the inlet flow direction is at right angles to the outlet flow. Very occasionally a mixed flow configuration is found, where a centrifugal impeller rotates within what appears to be an axial flow casing. If there is any doubt, and the fan identification plate is readable, a telephone call to the maker will confirm the type.

The type of drive describes the way the fan impeller is connected to the drive motor: either direct, where the impeller shaft is the same as that of the motor, or V-belt driven, where a pulley is attached to the fan shaft and another to the motor and V-shaped belts connect the two like a chain on a bicycle. The pulleys should always be covered with a guard, which may make counting the number of belts difficult. The fan diameter means the outside diameter of the rotating impeller and will be almost the same as the inlet duct diameter in the case of the axial flow fan and slightly larger than inlet duct diameter on the centrifugal type. Many of the centrifugal impellers are designed to be withdrawn through an opening in the casing of the inlet duct side, and an estimate of the diameter of that opening will indicate the diameter of the impeller.

The fan rotational speed will be the same as the motor speed with direct driven fans, and that can be read either from the identification plate of the motor or the fan casing. With V-belt driven fans it will be necessary to measure the speed by placing a portable tachometer on the end of the fan shaft and this may involve removing the guard: an operation that must be done with the fan stationary. The fan must then be started up and the shaft speed carefully measured, making sure that no part of the measurer's body or clothing can come into contact with the belts or pulleys. Ideally, arrangements should be made to have a small opening cut into the casing opposite the end of the fan shaft sufficiently large to allow the tip of the tachometer to be pushed into the shaft.

The direction of rotation is extremely important to note, particularly with fans driven by 3-phase electric motors. If the wiring to the motor has been connected incorrectly the motor will run in reverse. With axial flow fans this results in the air flowing in the opposite direction, and is usually quickly noticed and rectified, but with centrifugal fans the air continues to flow in the correct direction but at a greatly reduced flow rate. The direction of rotation needs to be described in relation to one side or the other of the fan. It is recommended that the fan be viewed from the side of the electric motor and described as 'clockwise' or 'anticlockwise'. If it is clockwise then the word 'anti' should be struck out on the form. Some fans have the correct direction marked on the casing, but if not the correct direction of a centrifugal fan can be deduced by observing the scroll shape of the fan casing. The impeller should rotate towards the expansion of the scroll.

The remaining information can usually be obtained from the label either on the motor or the fan casing.

The filter specifications – there are many types of filter to be found in industry, all variations of basic types: dry centrifugal (cyclones), electrostatic, fabric (bag or cartridge filters), wet scrubbers, absorbers, thermal oxidisers, catalytic cleaners. All that needs to be placed in the type box is one of these. The make and serial number can be obtained from the identification plate on the device. If it is a fabric filter the total surface area of the filtration medium is useful to have as a filter air velocity can be calculated from the volume flow rate.

The static pressure across the device, particularly if it is a fabric filter, will indicate the condition of the fabric, therefore it is useful to know what it should be when in good condition. If it is higher than normal it indicates blocked or partially blocked fabric; if it is below normal it will indicate either a hole in the fabric or a reduced flow rate for some other reason. By subtracting the static pressure at the filter outlet from that at the inlet the pressure across can be calculated. Static pressure at the inlet will indicate the condition of the ductwork system: if it is higher than normal it may indicate a blockage in the ductwork and if lower may indicate a reduced flow rate of the fan or a hole in the system.

Some systems have a secondary filter or a combination of two filters in series. There is provision for details of the second filter to be entered under the first.

Extract point specifications – here is an opportunity to enter details of the suction inlet, which can be one of several types, namely a glove box or total enclosure, a booth or chemical fume cupboard, a canopy hood, a side hood, a flexible arm moveable hood, or a slot. There is provision on the form to insert the face dimensions, duct diameter and area. Design operating conditions can be inserted in the columns for face velocity, duct velocity, volume flow rate and static pressure. There is space to qualify any of these in the comments column.

With regard to total enclosures such as glove boxes, air velocities and volume flow rates are not relevant and in any case may not be measurable. However, static pressure is important as it is the negative static pressure that prevents the pollutant being controlled from escaping.

The sketch – this need not be a detailed scale drawing but a schematic fine diagram showing all the relevant items making up the system. Duct sizes should be indicated and any measuring points numbered consecutively and marked on the diagram.

General – when a new ventilation plant is specified, pages 1 and 2 of this proforma can be handed to the supplier with a request to complete the details. The routine measurements that are recorded on pages 3 and 4 can be compared with those specified and a judgement made as to the success of the system.

Further reading

American Conference of Government Industrial Hygienists (1999) Testing of ventilation systems. In: *Industrial Ventilation* (23rd edn). ACGIH, Lansing, Michigan.

British Occupational Hygiene Society (1987) *Controlling Airborne Contaminants in the Workplace.* Technical Guide No. 7. Science Reviews Ltd, Leeds.

BSI Standards (1980) *Fans for General Purpose.* Part 1. Methods of testing performance. BS 848. BSI Standards, Milton Keynes.

Daly, B.B. (1979) *Woods Practical Guide to Fan Engineering.* Woods of Colchester, Colchester.

Gill, F.S. (1980) Ventilation. In: *Occupational Hygiene* (eds H.A. Waldron & J.M. Harrington), pp. 122–143. Blackwell Science, Oxford.

SI 1999/437 and Approved Code of Practice (1999) *Control of Substances Hazardous to Health Regulations.* HMSO, London.

Appendix

Record of ventilation plant (in accordance with COSHH Regulations) (page 1)

Name and address of company	
Department or site	
Location of plant	
Identification of plant	
Hazardous substances controlled by plant	
Type of plant (for sketch see page 2)	

Fan details: maker: serial no.			Fan Speed rpm anticlockwise (from drive side)	
Fan type (e.g. guide vane, bifurc, forward bladed, etc.) Axial dia mm centrif dia mm			Max design speed rpm	
Drive type (e.g. direct, V-belt, no. of belts)			Motor: maker speed rpm	
Duty: Volume flow rate $m^3\,s^{-1}$ Static or total press. Pa Air power kW			Voltage phase	
Inlet dia: mm Outlet dimens: mm			Full load current amp	

Primary air cleaner details: type:		Static press.	
Maker		inlet	Pa
Serial no:		outlet	Pa
Filter area:	m^2	across	Pa
Design volume flow	$m^3\,s^{-1}$	change at	Pa

Primary air cleaner details: type:		Static press.	
Maker		inlet	Pa
Serial no:		outlet	Pa
Filter area:	m^2	across	Pa
Design volume flow	$m^3\,s^{-1}$	change at	Pa

Record of ventilation plant (page 2)

Sketch of plant layout, label ventilation plant items and indicate measurement positions

Extract points, showing as far as possible the design values of performance (see sketch).

Point no.	Type (e.g. hood, booth, etc.)	Face dimensions mm	Duct dia. mm	Area m^2	Face vel. $m\ s^{-1}$	Duct vel. $m\ s^{-1}$	Flow rate. $m^3\ s^{-1}$	Stat. press. Pa	Comments

Results of routine ventilation measurements

Extract plant (hood, slot, enclosure, etc., see sketch and initial details on page 2)

Identification of plant:

Point	Date	Static press. Pa	Air velocity $m\ s^{-1}$	Volume flow $m^3\ s^{-1}$	Instrument used	Comments

Results of visual inspection and/or measurements

Describe below any defects found in any parts of the ventilation system and state what remedial action is required

Measurements/inspection made by Name:	Employer's name and address:

Air monitoring results as part of COSHH Reg. 9 Examination and Test
(state units e.g. mg m^{-3} or ppm)

Is exhaust air returned to workplace? yes/no
If yes, give below returned air concentrations (state substance and units, e.g. Xylene 450 mg m^{-3})

Date	Concentration	Date	Concentration	Date	Concentration

Are these concentrations satisfactory? yes/no If no, state remedial action required

Test point	Date	Duration	Subs.	Conc.	Subs.	Conc.	Subs.	Conc.	Subs.	Conc.
1										
2										
3										
4										
5										
6										
7										
8										
9										
10										
11										
12										
13										
14										
15										

Name of occupational hygienist or organisation
Do any of the results above show concentrations exceeding OES or MEL? yes/no If yes, give details

5 Noise

Introduction

In modern environments it is difficult to find a situation where noise does not occur. Even people in offices and computer rooms experience noise levels that may cause concern and many industrial situations are noted for their continuous sound output.

The production and transmission of sound is complex and its understanding involves a good knowledge of physics and mathematics. However, recent developments in instrumentation are such that people whose knowledge of acoustics is limited can now provide for themselves a good assessment of the acoustical environment in which people work. Expert advice need now only be required if noise levels require reduction or a process is to be designed with minimum noise output.

In order to assess the health hazard of a noisy working environment it is necessary to measure the 'dose' of noise to which the worker becomes exposed or receives. This means assessing the sound intensity, the duration of exposure and the pitch of the sounds produced in the work place.

On the first day of January 1990 the Noise at Work Regulations of 1989 came into force. In them, three action levels are defined: the 'first' is a dose level of daily personal noise exposure ($L_{EP,d}$) of 85 dB(A) and the 'second' an $L_{EP,d}$ of 90 dB(A). Another is a 'peak action level' of 200 Pa (140 dB) and refers to a single event not to be exceeded. Certain courses of action are to be taken if the noise dose reaches the first, second or the peak levels.

Sound is produced at a range of pitches from a very low rumble or hum to a very high-pitched squeal or hiss. The pitch is termed 'frequency' and is expressed in hertz (Hz). This is the number of vibrations or pressure waves per second. The lowest pitch sound that can be heard by the human ear of a healthy young person is at about 20 Hz and the highest up to 18 000 Hz (18 kHz). Each time the frequency is doubled the note will rise one octave. Middle C on the piano is 256 Hz and C an octave above is 512 Hz. The ear is most sensitive to the frequencies of between 500 Hz and 4 kHz of which 500 Hz–2 kHz is the frequency of speech. Unless a sound is a pure tone, which is unusual, most noises are made up of sounds of many frequencies and intensities and when assessing the intensity it may be necessary to discover what they are over the whole range of frequencies, that is, to measure the sound spectrum. For convenience it is usual to divide the sounds into octave bands and use a measuring instrument that assesses the intensities of all notes between the octaves and express it as a mid-octave intensity. The mid-octave frequencies chosen for this analysis are: 62.5 Hz, 125 Hz, 250 Hz, 500 Hz, 1 kHz, 2 kHz, 4 kHz, 8 kHz, and sometimes 16 kHz. Thus a spectrum of a noise will quote the intensities at each of these mid-octave band frequencies. A technique for measuring a noise spectrum is given later.

Sound is pressure changes in the air, which are picked up by the ear drum and transmitted to the brain. The pressure is normally measured in Newtons per square metre or Pascal (Pa). The quietest sound that can be heard is at about 0.00002 Pa (20 μPa), but at 25 m from a jet aircraft taking off it is 200 Pa, which is 10^7 times greater. The intensity of sound is expressed in a unit known as the 'decibel' (dB), which is a convenient way of expressing a value that can have an extremely wide range.

The decibel compares the sound pressure being measured with the pressure at the threshold of hearing and, because the range of pressures found in acoustics is so large, is expressed on a log scale (to base 10). It is mathematically defined as:

$$dB = 20 \log_{10}\left(\frac{P_a}{P_r}\right)$$

where P_a = the sound pressure of the sound being considered, and

P_r = the reference sound pressure at the threshold of hearing, that is, 0.00002 Pa.

To illustrate this, Table 5.1 indicates typical everyday sound levels. Because the measurement of decibels is on a log scale, one sound is approximately twice as loud as the other when the difference between the two is 3 dB. If two sounds are emitted at the same time their combined intensity is not the numerical sum of each separate intensity but must be added according to Fig. 5.1.

Table 5.1. Typical sound intensities

		Sound intensities	
	Pressure (Pa)	Bel (B)	Decibel (dB)
Threshold of hearing	0.00002	0	0
Quiet office	0.002	4	40
Ringing alarm clock at 1 m	0.2	8	80
Ship's engine room	20	12	120
Turbo-jet engine	2000	16	160

Example: two sounds at 90 dB each will combine to have an intensity of 93 dB; one at 90 and one at 92 will combine to an intensity of 94; one at 90 and one at 100 will combine to be 100; that is, if two sounds are ten or more decibels different, then the lower intensity will not be added.

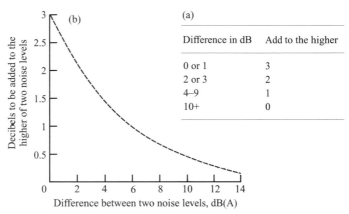

Fig. 5.1. (a) Simplified method for adding decibel levels. (b) Chart adding two unequal noise levels.

Weighting

As noise is a combination of sounds at various frequencies and intensities, the noise intensity can be either expressed as a spectrum, mentioned previously, or as a combination of all frequencies summed together in one value. As the human ear is more sensitive to certain frequencies than others, it is possible to make allowances for that in the electronic circuitry of a sound level meter. That is, certain frequencies are suppressed as others are boosted in order to approximate to the response of the ear.

This technique is known as weighting and there are A, B, C and D weightings available for various purposes. The one that is most usually quoted is the A weighting because it mimics the response of the human ear, and instruments measuring sound intensity with that weighting give readings in dB(A). However, dB(C) is becoming the more favoured scale. The weighting given to the mid-octave band frequencies for the A and C scales is given in Table 5.2.

When assessing an employee's exposure to noise it is the dose that is important, that is, the duration of exposure in relation to the noise intensity that needs to be taken into account. This is simple if the noise produced is constant throughout the period of exposure.

Table 5.2. Mid-octave band frequency corrections for dB(A) weighting

Frequency (Hz)	62.5	125	250	500	1000	2000	4000	8000
Correction for dB(A)	-26	-16	-9	-3	0	$+1$	$+1$	-1
Correction for dB(C)	-1	0	0	0	0	0	-1	-3

It is then a matter of measuring the level and noting the time when the worker entered the area and when he or she left. However, most workplace noise fluctuates as different operations take place and various items of noise-producing equipment or machinery are turned on or off. Also, impact noise such as hammering, riveting and pressing cause short duration peaks of high intensity. Thus it is not easy to establish how long an employee has been exposed to each noise to work out a total dose.

The unit of L_{eq} is used to express noise dose. It is defined as the equivalent continuous noise level that would give the same total amount of sound energy as the fluctuating noise. It is, in effect, a time-weighted average noise energy of the peaks and troughs of exposure over the period of time under consideration. Sound level meters are available that will record L_{eq} and give the duration over which it was measured (Fig. 5.2).

Equipment available

Sound level meters

Essentially a sound level meter consists of a microphone that converts the sound waves to electrical impulses, some electronic circuitry that modifies and amplifies the signal according to the demands of the user, and an output section to display the signal in units of sound as required. Portable sound level meters are battery powered, thus the battery charge condition must also be displayed. The quality of sound level meter is governed by the requirements of several British Standards notably BS5969, BS6698. Meters are graded according to their accuracy from type 0 to type 3 as shown in Table 5.3. With most sound level meters the difference between type 1 and type 2 is the quality of the microphone, the electronics being the same. Therefore for everyday use it is wise to buy a type 2 meter and when more precision is required a type 1 microphone can be added.

Table 5.3. Typical accuracy of meters used for measuring industrial noise (BS5969)

BS/IEC grade	Typical use	Amplitude range on a single setting (dB)	Typical overall accuracy
0	Laboratory reference	70	± 0.5
1	Laboratory and field	60	± 1.0
2	General field	50	± 1.5
3	Field survey	50	± 3.0

The facilities offered start at a simple noise meter that just indicates dB(A) but others can provide a wide range of displays such as L_{eq}, octave and third octave band analysers (Fig. 5.3), real-time spectral analysers, data loggers and many other useful facilities. The quality and facilities that a sound level meter offers is reflected in its cost. Prices start at around £400 for the simplest instruments and rise to

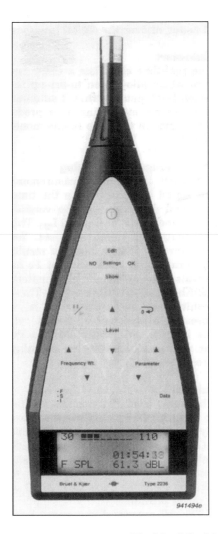

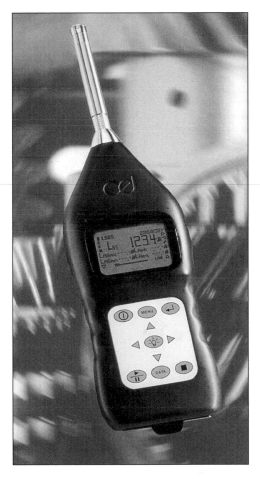

Fig. 5.2. *(left)* Modular precision sound level meter (Bruel and Kjaer UK Ltd).

Fig. 5.3. *(right)* Sound level meter with octave band analyser (CEL Instruments Ltd).

several thousand pounds for the most precise ones having a wide range of facilities.

Recent work has shown that impulse noise and short-term transient peaks of sound have an important effect upon noise exposure. Most traditional sound level meters do not have sufficient dynamic range or a fast enough response time to correctly record these short-term events. International standards now specify requirements for impulse precision sound level meters that respond very quickly. The most recently developed meters comply with the new standards but older designs which are still on the market do not. Care should be taken when purchasing new instruments to ensure that the type is suitable for the purpose required.

Weight and size also vary, the ones having the most facilities being the heaviest and most bulky. Where important decisions are to be made based on noise measurements or if legal arguments are to be based on results, then the precision grade (type 1) instrument must be used, preferably handled by an experienced and qualified person.

Noise dosimeters

The sheer size and weight of a meter that has a noise dose facility precludes its use for personal measurement. Therefore, small noise dosimeters are available that can be easily carried by an employee throughout the shift and which will not hinder the task to be performed. These will sense all noise levels to which they are exposed making a record against time and storing the information for retrieval on demand. Dosimeters can either have an integral microphone, the whole unit designed to be worn in the breast pocket, or they can have a separate microphone that can be clipped to the lapel with a lead carrying the signal to a small box containing the battery and electronics, which can be carried in a pocket or hung on a belt. An example of a noise dosimeter is shown in Fig. 5.4. Some dosimeters can be used as an integrating sound level meter by replacing the microphone and associated cable designed to be placed on the lapel with a mast on which a microphone is placed.

As with sound level meters, noise dosimeters can be either of precision or industrial grade. Some are available as data loggers with facilities that can provide statistical analysis of the recorded sound levels and some can feed information into microcomputers for further analysis (Fig. 5.5).

Calibration

In order to check that the meter is reading correctly it is necessary to have a source of sound of a known intensity and frequency that can be introduced through the microphone, excluding all other sounds except the calibration tone. All meters have an adjusting screw, which can be turned to make the display read the intensity of the calibrator.

Most calibrators for portable meters are battery powered, producing the calibration tone electronically. They must be of a tight fit around the microphone of the meter to ensure no other sounds are being received at the same time. To this end rubber O-rings are used as seals and some have adapters to fit various microphone sizes. Calibration tones vary in intensity from one manufacturer to another although 94 dB at 1000 Hz is the most usual. If

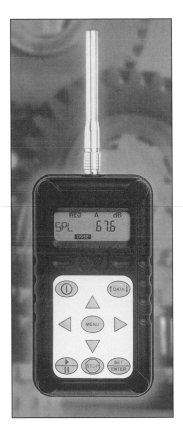

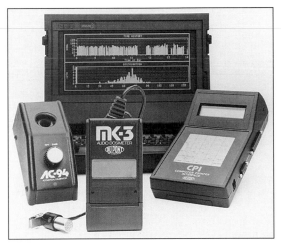

Fig. 5.4. *(left)* Personal ISO noise dosimeter (CEL Instruments).

Fig. 5.5. *(right)* Metrosonics audio dosimeter (Shaw City Ltd).

dB(A) scales are to be checked then they must be at a frequency of 1000 Hz. There is a calibrator available known as a 'piston-phone', which produces a tone of 124 dB at 250 Hz, and this is suitable for calibrating an octave band analyser at that frequency.

It is important to check the meter regularly with the calibrator and at least once before starting a series of readings or at the start of a working shift. It is also important to ensure that the calibrator battery is in good order. Each manufacturer gives instructions as to how to achieve this. Calibrators need to be returned to the manufacturer from time to time for servicing and re-calibration.

To measure a steady workroom noise

Aim

Workroom noise produced from machines or items of equipment can be a source of irritation, stress and/or can lead to hearing damage. It is important to be able to measure noise levels at various workplaces to establish whether it is necessary to take remedial action to control the employees' exposure and to identify the main sources of noise, as required in the UK by the Noise at Work Regulations, 1989. Following on from that it may be necessary to designate certain areas of the factory as hearing conservation areas in which people are forbidden to enter without wearing suitable protection.

Equipment required

A sound level meter having a dB(A) weighting capability (for example, Bruel & Kjaer, Fig. 5.2), a calibration device suitable for the microphone on the meter, that is, of the same diameter to ensure a good fit, a small screwdriver, a tripod capable of holding the meter may also be useful but is not essential.

Method

Before commencing please check the manufacturer's instructions. The steps described below do not apply to any specific instrument but may be included in manufacturers' instructions.

1 Check the battery output by switching on the 'battery test' switch. Each manufacturer has its own method of indicating the battery charge condition, as shown in their instruction manual. The position of the test switch varies for different instruments but is usually associated with the power on/off switch and is always clearly marked. If the batteries do not have sufficient power they should be replaced. It is wise to test the battery before leaving for the survey unless charged spares are carried.

2 Switch on the instrument and allow it to warm up for at least 2 minutes.

3 Calibrate the instrument as follows: remove the microphone cover, fit the calibrator over the microphone and set the scale to dB(A) and to the correct range* for the output of the calibrator. If the instrument has a 'fast' and 'slow' response switch set it to 'fast'. Turn on the calibrator and observe the reading on the meter. If it does not read exactly the calibration value adjust the

---

* Meters vary in the way they indicate the reading: some show a value on a dial to add to or subtract from the setting of a range switch; some indicate directly on a dial according to the range to which it is switched and some give a digital readout of actual decibels.

needle by turning the calibration screw using the small screwdriver. The adjusting screw will be labelled in a variety of ways, e.g. 'Adj', 'Gain Adj' or 'CAL'.

4   To measure the noise exposure remove the microphone cap, turn on, switch to 'fast' response and hold the instrument at arm's length away from the body keeping it at least 1 m above the floor. If an individual worker's exposure is to be measured hold the microphone close to each ear of the worker but pointing towards the source and note the reading on each side. If the meter is fluctuating too much to obtain a readable value then switch it to 'slow' response and read again. If the needle rises above or falls below the range (see footnote, page 132) of the meter, switch the range control to the appropriate value. In order to minimise the sound-blocking effect of the measurer's body, mount the instrument on a tripod if one is available and stand at least 0.5 m away from it when reading the meter. Some instruments have their microphone on a length of cable so that it can be mounted away from the meter for this very purpose.

5   If the worker is at a noisy machine it may be useful to obtain a background noise, therefore repeat step 4 above with the machine switched off. If there is little difference in the noise level between the background only, and the machine plus the background (i.e. less than 3 dB), then other sources of noise may be just as important.

Results

From the results obtained it may be possible to establish whether employees are subjected to noise levels exceeding those defined in local statutes: for example, the UK Noise at Work Regulations, or the EEC Noise Directive 1986. If the noise is steady above 85 dB(A) and the worker is present most of the day, certain actions have to be taken as defined in those statutes. It should be remembered that even if these levels are not exceeded annoyance and stress can be induced and some people are susceptible to levels below that.

To measure the spectrum of a continuous noise by octave band analysis

Aim

In order to ascertain the range of frequencies represented in a problematical workroom noise it is necessary to break that noise down into bands of pitch and to measure the intensity of each band. In this way it is possible to establish what frequencies in the spectrum are the loudest so that the effect of the noise can be assessed. For example, if the loudest sounds are in the speech frequencies

(500 Hz–2 kHz) it will be clear that speech communication will be difficult or impossible, and if the loudest sounds are at the higher frequencies of 1–6 kHz then those people exposed to it are more likely to suffer temporary or permanent hearing damage than if the lower pitches are represented. From this information the acoustic engineer can decide what remedial action needs to be taken as different spectra require different attenuation techniques to reduce the levels. It is generally easier to suppress high-frequency sounds than low rumbles or hums, which, although they are less damaging to hearing, are nevertheless extremely irritating, particularly if they continue for long periods of time. Also, from the spectrum, if hearing defenders are to be prescribed then the type most suited to the noise characteristic can be specified.

Equipment required

A precision sound level meter with an octave band filter set incorporated (for example, CEL, Fig. 5.3) or added (a third octave band instrument could also be used to provide more information but is more expensive and less common); a calibration device suitable for the microphone on the meter, that is, of the same diameter to ensure a good fit; and a small screwdriver. A tripod capable of holding the meter may also be useful but is not essential.

Method

1   Check the battery output by switching on the 'battery test' switch. The position of the test switch varies for different instruments but is usually associated with the power on/off switch and is always clearly marked. If the indicator fails to reach the level the batteries should be replaced. It is wise to test the battery before leaving for the survey unless fully charged spares are carried.

2   Switch on the instrument and allow it to warm up for at least 2 minutes.

3   Calibrate the instrument as follows: remove the microphone cover, fit the calibrator over the microphone and set the instrument to 'Ext filter' or 'Filter' and set the response to 'fast'. Select the meter range (see footnote, page 132) to the correct one for the output of the calibrator. On the filter set, switch the octave band selector to the frequency of the calibrator. Turn on the calibrator and observe the reading on the meter. If it does not read exactly the calibration value adjust the needle or digital display by turning the calibration screw using the small screwdriver. The adjuster will be labelled in a variety of ways, e.g. 'Adj', 'Gain Adj' or 'CAL'.

4   Locate the position where the measurements are required to be taken. This may be at the place where the worker is stationed

or, if the point of maximum noise level is required, then it will be necessary to ascertain this by using the dB(A) scale as described previously, and measuring in various places in the workroom until this point is established.

5   To obtain the sound spectrum: remove the microphone cover, turn on the instrument, switch to 'Ext filter' or 'Filter' and to 'slow' response and hold the instrument at arm's length away from the body, pointing towards the noise source. Turn the external filter band selection switch to 62.5 Hz and note the reading. If the scale on the meter is at the wrong range select the correct one (see footnote, page 132).

Repeat for each filter band setting up to 8 kHz. In order to minimise the shielding effect of the observer's body the instrument can be mounted on a tripod and read from a distance of at least 0.5 m.

6   As a check, turn off the external filter and set the instrument to dB(A) and measure the A weighting level.

Results

Plot the results obtained from the measurement on a copy of the noise rating (NR) curves given in Fig. 5.6. Join up the points with straight lines (not a smooth curve). Examine the shape of the spectrum to establish whether there is a steady output at all frequencies or whether certain frequencies predominate. It is beyond the scope of this text to provide ways of judging the results as the field of acoustics is very specialised. The reader is advised to seek further advice by perusing a good acoustics text or by consulting an acoustician with experience in the field of human response to noise. Nevertheless, the NR curves are given to provide some guidance. The noise rating of the spectrum obtained can be said to be the same as the curve immediately above the highest point on the spectrum drawn – see the example in Fig. 5.6.

The dB(A) of the spectrum can be obtained by adding the intensity of adjacent bands corrected for dB(A) until a single value is obtained. Addition of sound levels is quickly but approximately done using Fig. 5.1. Draw up a record sheet as shown in the example in Table 5.4 and write the results on the second line.

Example

With several machines running in a duplicating room in an office building a sound spectrum was obtained as shown in the second line of Table 5.4. The measured dB(A) level was 82. The sound spectrum is plotted on the NR curves shown as a broken line.

The calculated dB(A) agrees with the measured value. It can be seen that the plotted spectrum lies just below the NR80 curve, the inference being that this is a very high noise level to be experienced

Table 5.4. Record sheet for calculation of A-weighted decibel values

Octave band mid-frequency (Hz)	63	125	250	500	1000	2000	4000	8000
Measured levels (dB)	65	74	76	78	78	75	72	67
Correction for dB(A)	−26	−16	−9	−3	0	+1	+1	−1
Result	39	58	67	75	78	76	73	66

Addition from Fig. 5.1.

58   76   80   74

76   81

82 dB(A)

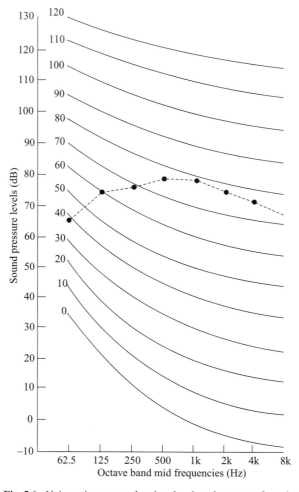

Fig. 5.6. Noise rating curves showing the plotted spectrum from the sample.

in an office situation and is above what might be desirable in an industrial workplace.

Recommended noise ratings

Broadcasting or recording studio	NR 15
Concert hall or a 500-seat theatre	NR 20
Class room, music room, TV studio, large conference room, bedroom	NR 25
Small conference room, library, church, cinema, courtroom	NR 30
Private office	NR 40
Restaurant	NR 45
General office with typewriters	NR 50
Workshop	NR 65

To measure the L_{eq} of a fluctuating workroom noise

Aim

The meaning of L_{eq} is explained on page 128 but essentially it is the equivalent steady level in dB(A) of a fluctuating noise over a period of time. It is used to establish the risk to which an employee is exposed when subjected to a continually changing noise over the course of a working period. From the result it will be possible to decide whether or not action is required to be taken to reduce the exposure by reducing the noise intensity, reducing the duration of exposure, or providing some form of hearing protection.

Equipment required

An integrating sound level meter, a calibrating device suitable for the microphone on the meter, that is, of the same diameter to ensure a good fit, a small screwdriver, and a tripod capable of holding the meter are needed.

Method

1   Check the battery output by switching on the 'battery test' switch. The position of the test switch varies for different instruments but is usually associated with the power on/off switch and is always clearly marked. If the indicator fails to reach the required level the batteries should be replaced. It is wise to test the battery before leaving for the survey unless fully charged spares are carried.

2   Switch on the instrument and allow it to warm up for at least 2 minutes.

3   Calibrate the instrument according to manufacturer's instructions.

4   Locate the instrument in the position where the measurements are required to be taken, which would normally be at a work station or close to an employee. Because it is to be left for a period of time it is necessary to mount it on a tripod or on some vibration-free surface. After ensuring that the meter is turned on, the microphone cover removed and the weighting switch at 'A', switch to L_{eq} at the moment when the worker's exposure to the noise starts.

5   At the end of the period note the value of the L_{eq} as displayed. Some instruments show this continuously throughout the test period but others require a display button to be pressed to provide a digital readout at any time during the test. Most instruments display the duration of the test period in hours when the 'elapsed time' button is pushed.

Results

Standards of continuous noise or its equivalent energy, L_{eq}, that are set to reduce hearing damage vary from one country to another. In the Great Britain the second 'action level' defined under the Noise at Work Regulations 1989 (see page 125) is regarded as a 100 per cent dose. Thus if a noise dosimeter records over 100 per cent it shows that this action level has been exceeded. Table 5.5 shows various noise levels and durations of exposure, all of which represent 100 per cent dose.

The use of a personal noise dosimeter

In order to assess the degree of auditory hazard to which an employee is exposed during the course of his or her job it is useful to monitor the worker rather than the workplace. This is particularly so if the worker moves about into various levels of noise exposure or where the use of a bulky integrating sound level meter is difficult or impossible due to the nature of the operations taking place. Personal dosimeters are designed to be socially acceptable and cause minimal interference when worn, as they are small and light in weight.

Equipment required

A noise dosimeter, a calibration device suitable for the dosimeter, and a small screwdriver are needed.

Table 5.5.   Noise dosages representing 100 per cent for UK dosimeters

Limiting dB(A)	Maximum duration of exposure
90	8 h
93	4 h
96	2 h
99	1 h
102	30 min
105	15 min
108	7 min
111	4 min
114	2 min
117	1 min
120	30 s

Method

Dosimeters from different manufacturers are so widely different that it is not possible to be general in describing their use. Therefore the reader is advised to follow closely the instructions provided with the instrument. However, some general comments are provided here for the guidance of users.

1   The readout displays of dosimeters vary. Some types give a numerical digital display using liquid crystal diodes but other models use a binary code display involving sixteen lights arranged in groups of four, each group representing: units, tens, hundreds and thousands. The instruction books give guidance on the interpretation of the display.

The result of the measurement is expressed as a percentage of the allowed daily L_{eq} exposure, thus an exposure of 90 dB(A) for 8 hours would be 100 per cent, as would 93 dB(A) measured for 4 hours or 96 for 2 hours. Formulae and conversion charts are given in the handbooks to convert the recorded percentage to L_{eq} after taking into account the duration of the test. Also some meters display a peak level warning that indicates when a specified dB(A) value has been exceeded during the test.

2   Switching of the meter is designed to provide protection and to make the device as tamper-proof as possible. This is achieved in a variety of ways. In one model the instrument is turned on or off and the display actuated by depressing microswitches set below the level of the cover by poking a narrow allen key through holes in the casing. In another model these operations are actuated by magnetically operated reed switches, a magnet being provided for the purpose, whilst a third type has all its switches and displays hidden by a sliding cover. This can be sealed by an adhesive label which indicates whether the seal has been disturbed.

3   As a dosimeter is a device which stores information over a period of time it is important to ensure that all previous measurements are cleared from the memory. Thus a re-setting procedure must be adopted if the readout is not showing zero.

4   The instrument must be calibrated before use as directed by the manufacturer.

5   The microphone should be placed as close to the ear as possible, either by clipping it to the lapel or by attaching it to the rim of a helmet. It should be noted that one ear of the worker may be exposed to a louder noise than the other and in this event the microphone should be attached on that side of the worker's body. Care should be taken to ensure that the microphone is not knocked in any way in the course of the worker's actions as artificially high readings may result. Microphones should also be protected by a dust cover when in use, although it is necessary to remove it when calibrating.

Results

After converting the displayed percentage to a true worker exposure a judgement can be made as to the likely harmful effects using Table 5.4. If necessary, action should be taken to minimise worker exposure to the noise. Control should be at source rather than using hearing protection.

Possible problems

Employees find that being asked to wear a noise dosimeter is a novelty; their colleagues are also intrigued by the device. There is a desire to tamper with the instrument by shouting into it or, worse, by removing the microphone from the lapel to hold it close to a noisy machine. These actions render the results useless. Unless close supervision is applied this is likely to occur on the first or even the second day of a survey. By the third day the novelty has worn off and results will be more reliable.

To determine the degree of noise exposure and the actions to take

Using the techniques described above and by following the algorithm shown in Fig. 5.7, it is possible to delineate areas to be labelled as ear protection zones and determine whether further action is required to comply with local noise regulations. The actions set out below follow the algorithm and are modelled on the UK Noise at Work Regulations.

Action 1   set the meter to dB(A) and measure noise level

Action 2   question: are the levels above 85 dB(A)?
                if no, record it and take no further action
                if yes, estimate $L_{EP,d}$

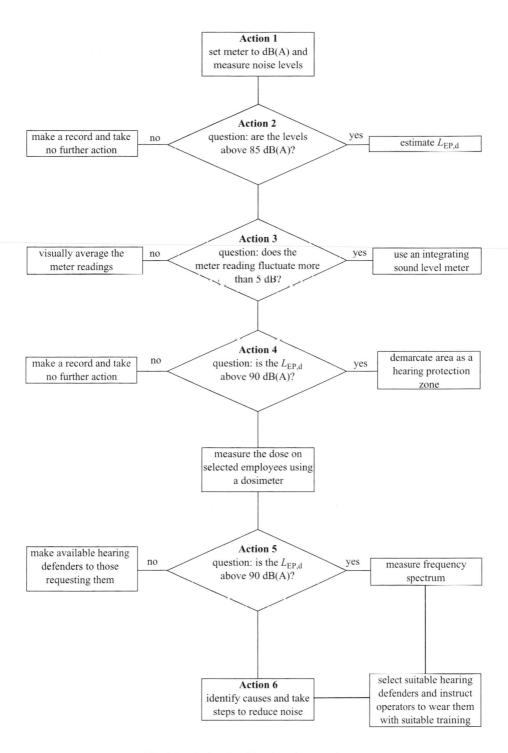

Fig. 5.7. Action algorithm for noise control.

Action 3	question: does the meter reading fluctuate more than 5 dB?
	if no, visually average the meter readings
	if yes, use an integrating sound level meter
Action 4	question: is the $L_{EP,d}$ above 90 dB(A)?
	if no, make a record
	if yes, demarcate area as a hearing protection zone and measure the dose on selected employees using a dosimeter
Action 5	question: is the $L_{EP,d}$ above 90 dB(A)?
	if no, make available hearing defenders to those requesting them
	if yes, measure frequency spectrum, select suitable hearing defenders and instruct operators to wear them with suitable training
Action 6	identify causes and take steps to reduce noise

To measure the triaxial vibration on a hand-held tool: the Castle method

Hand–arm vibration syndrome is a widely known industrial disease affecting thousands of employees. It causes pain to the sufferer and results in the loss of ability to grip properly. One of its manifestations is the disease known as vibration-induced white finger, VWF. Typical operations that may lead to the disease are the use of the following types of hand-held tools: percussive hammers, percussive concrete breakers, portable grinders, chain saws, circular saws, grass cutters, strimmers and many others. The disease is reportable under the Reporting of Injuries, Diseases and Dangerous Occurrences Regulations 1985 (RIDDOR) and is a prescribed disease.

A tool can vibrate in three directions along axes at right angles to each other described as x, y and z. The frequency of vibration can vary between 2 and 1500 Hz but is most damaging at 5 to 20 Hz. The hazard to health is usually judged by the average (root mean square) acceleration measured in m s^{-2} using an instrument having a frequency weighting network. As with noise, it is the 'dose' of vibration that causes the damage, therefore the employees' dose has to be adjusted to a reference period of 8 hours. The instrument that measures the acceleration is known as an accelerometer.

Most accelerometers measure only along one axis but the Castle GA2001 Vibration and HARM® (Hand Arm Risk Measurement) instrument is capable of collecting and processing the signals along three axes by using three accelerometers attached to a triaxial accelerometer mounting block. This block can be gripped between the operator's hand and the handle of the vibration machine. In this way the block will move in tandem with the operator's hand thus

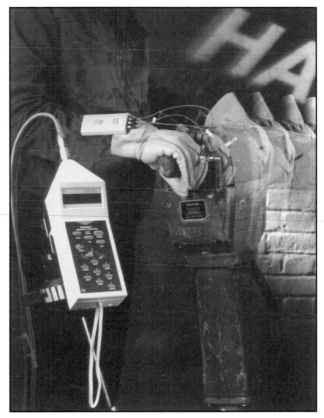

Fig. 5.8. The GA2001 Castle HARM0 Vibration Meter (Castle Group Limited).

reproducing the movement experienced. The measuring instrument is also capable of analysing the results and calculating the 8-hour dose.

Equipment required
Castle GA2001 octave band vibration and HARM® meter, three KD1004 industrial accelerometers each fitted with ZL1094 accelerometer cables, KD1209 HARM® BLOK hand-held accelerometer block, KD1301 Tri-Axial interface, portable printer (optional), mounting tripod (optional).

Method
1   Ask the machine operator to prepare their normal task and to inform you of how long any operation takes and how many times during a normal 8-hour shift this operation occurs. From this it will be possible to estimate the total running time of the vibrating tool during the course of the shift.

2 Fit the accelerometers to the mounting block and connect the three tri-axial cables to the KD1301 interface. This unit can be strapped to the operator's lower arm using the Velcro strap.

3 Connect the triaxial interface cable to the top of the GA2001 meter by lining up the red dots: it is a push fit, *do not twist*.

4 Ask the operator to hold the mounting block between two fingers so that the foot plate makes good contact with the handle of the vibrating tool. Note that with two-handed machines both hands may have to be tested in turn.

5 Switch on the GA2001 by pushing the power button for at least 2 seconds.

6 Press the HARM button once and wait until the meter has passed through a series of self checks. When ready, a display thus: HARM > CURRENT RECORD will be shown on the screen. Note the two arrows pointing inwards toward the word CURRENT.

7 Press the right-hand arrow to select > RECORD (note the two arrows are now pointing inwards towards the word RECORD). Press ENTER.

8 At this stage there is a a choice between MANUAL and AUTO. The manual mode allows the measurer to select the measuring duration during the logging process in each axis. The auto allows the user to pre-determine the measurement duration along each axis (typically 10–30 seconds is chosen to ensure that the measuring period is representative). Initially it is advisable to select manual until user experience has been gained. Select MANUAL and press ENTER.

9 The meter will ask for an employee identification number from 001–250: enter a number using the keypad and press ENTER. The display will show X-AXIS and the instantaneous vibration level, but as the operator has not started his/her task this value has no relevance.

10 Ask the operator to commence work with the vibrating tool.

11 Allow the reading to stabilise and press ENTER.

12 After a suitable duration (typically 10–30 seconds) press ENTER. The display will now show Y-AXIS.

13 Repeat steps 10–12 for Y and Z axes.

14 The meter will now ask for exposure time by displaying EXPOSURE TIME. Enter the typical daily duration of exposure in hours and minutes as given by the operator in step 1 above. With the keypad press the duration in hours and press ENTER then press the duration in minutes and press ENTER.

15 The meter will now display as step 6 above, i.e. HARM > CURRENT < RECORD. At this stage the operation can be repeated for the same operator – for example, with the mounting block in the other hand – or for another operator.

16   When ready to retrieve the results press the right-hand arrow twice to display VIEW, then press ENTER. The display will ask for the employee number, which should be pressed in from the keypad followed by ENTER.

17   The display will now show time and date of each measurement. Use the right or left arrows to select the result required and press ENTER. This will display the X-axis acceleration (a_x). To obtain the results from the Y and Z axes press the right-hand arrow in turn. One more press of the right hand arrow will display the vector sum, i.e. $\sqrt{a_x{}^2 + a_y{}^2 + a_z{}^2}$. This is the average vibration experienced by the operator's hand over the measurement period.

18   To obtain an estimated 8-hour time-weighted average, taking into account the operator's estimation of total duration of use of the tool over the working day, press the right-hand arrow once more. This can be compared with the recommended action level of 2.8 m s^{-1} given in the HSE publication HS(G)88, Hand-arm Vibration.

Possible problems

If the wrong buttons have been pushed on the keypad it is possible to return to the HARM menu (as described in step 6 above) by pressing the vertical arrow.

Further reading

BSI Standards (1981) *Specification for Sound Level Meters.* BS 5969. BSI Standards, Milton Keynes.

Burns, W. (1973) *Noise and Man.* Murray, London.

Gardiner, K. (1995) Noise. In: *Occupational Hygiene* (eds H.A. Waldron & J.M. Harrington), pp. 123–150. Blackwell Science, Oxford.

Health and Safety Executive (1989) *Noise at Work. Guidance on Regulations.* HMSO, London.

Health and Safety Executive (1994) *Guidance HS(G)88: Hand-arm Vibration.* HSE Books, Sudbury, Suffolk.

King, I.J. (1980) Noise and vibration. In: *Occupational Hygiene* (eds H.A. Waldron & J.M. Harrington), pp. 144–194. Blackwell Scientific Publications, Oxford.

Sharland, I. (1979) *Practical Guide to Noise Control.* Woods of Colchester, Colchester.

SI 1989/1790 *Noise at Work Regulations, 1989.* HMSO, London.

Taylor, R. (1975) *Noise.* Penguin, New York (Pelican Books).

Webb, D.J. (ed.) (1976) *Noise Control in Industry.* Sound Research Laboratories, Colchester.

6 Light

Introduction

It is important that workplace lighting is maintained at an acceptable standard, that is, lighting levels must be sufficiently high to enable employees to see their tasks clearly, but not so high as to cause glare or dazzle. Poor workplace lighting not only creates eye strain, particularly if the task to be performed contains small detail, but can also cause fatigue leading to errors in the work and an increased accident risk. In the United Kingdom there is a legal requirement to 'provide every workplace with suitable and sufficient lighting' (Workplace Health, Safety and Welfare Regulations 1992). Therefore, it is important to be able to assess lighting levels in workplaces.

Sources of illumination can be divided into two: natural (daylight) and artificial (usually by means of electric lamps). Very few workplaces rely solely upon daylight whereas many are entirely artificially illuminated. Different levels of illumination are required for different tasks, thus workplace lighting must be designed for the type of work to be undertaken. Unfortunately, work patterns change and sources of illumination deteriorate with age, particularly in industrial situations: that is, windows and light fittings accumulate dirt, which reduces the amount of light emitted and surfaces become dirty, reducing the amount of light reflected from them. This often occurs so gradually that it goes unnoticed. Therefore, it is prudent for workplace lighting levels to be measured from time to time and the results checked against recommended standards.

However, it must be stressed that the presence of the correct level of illumination does not necessarily mean that the workplace is properly lit. The position of the source of light in relation to the worker and the workpiece may seriously affect the way the task is seen. The appearance of solid objects will be influenced by the direction from which the light comes and unshielded sources of light will cause glare if they appear within the field of view. Also, if the work involves the identification of different-coloured materials then certain sources of light can alter colours, sometimes making two different colours appear the same.

Units used in lighting

Luminous intensity. Symbol I, unit candela (Cd), which is the power of a source to emit light.

146

Luminous flux. Symbol Φ, unit lumen (lm), which is the luminous flux emitted within unit solid angle (one steradian) by a point source having a uniform luminous intensity of one candela. A lamp of one candela emits 4π lumens.

Illuminance. Symbol E, unit lux (or lumen m^{-2}), which is the luminous flux density at a surface. This is the unit that is used to express the lighting levels in a workroom.

Luminance. Symbol L, unit candela m^{-2}, which is the intensity of light emitted in a given direction by a unit area of luminous or reflecting surface.

Reflectance of a surface. Symbol R, dimensionless, which is the ratio of the flux reflected from a surface to the flux incident upon it.

Daylight factor. Symbol *DF*. Where daylight passing through windows is used to illuminate an indoor workplace, less than one-tenth of the outside light is likely to reach that place, and that amount decreases with distance from the window. When determining the lighting levels designed for the room, it is useful to compare the inside illuminance due to daylight with that prevailing outside at the same time on a percentage basis. For this purpose a value known as the 'daylight factor' is used, which is defined in Great Britain as the percentage of daylight illumination at a given point on a plane in a building relative to that simultaneously prevailing outside under an unobstructed, uniformly overcast sky. It is expressed mathematically as:

$$DF = \frac{E_i}{E_o} \times 100 \text{ per cent}$$

where E_i = the illuminance at a point inside, and

E_o = the simultaneous illumination outside.

The daylight factor at a point in a room is constant being dependent upon the solid angle subtended to the sky as viewed through the window or windows. Thus, once the daylight factor of a point in a room is determined it is always possible to predict its illumination level knowing the outside illuminance at a particular time by rearranging the above expression:

$$E_i = \frac{DF \text{ (per cent)} \times E_o}{100} \text{ (lumen m}^{-2}\text{)}$$

In south-east England the monthly average outside illumination at noon in July is 34 000 lux and at the same time in December is 7800 lux. The standard taken for the average exterior illuminance in this country is 5000 lux, thus when such a level occurs, a daylight factor of 1% at a point inside a building would produce an average of 50 lux (1% of 5000).

Diversity factor. This describes how even the distribution of light is in a room and is normally expressed as the minimum illuminance divided by the mean illuminance.

Utilisation factor. Symbol *UF*, unit lumen watt^{-1}, which indicates how effective the sources of artificial light are in relation to the total amount of power provided by the lamps. It is calculated from:

mean room illuminance (artificial light only)

$$(\text{lux}) \times UF = \frac{\text{area of floor (m}^2)}{\text{total wattage of lamps}}$$

Maintenance factor. Symbol *MF*. This indicates the condition of the lamps in relation to the amount of output the lamps produce based upon the utilisation factor. It is a value that will decrease as the lamps age or become dirty. It is calculated from the expression:

$$MF = \frac{\text{illuminance} \times \text{floor area}}{UF \times \text{total wattage of lamps}}.$$

Equipment available

Photometers

These are photoelectric devices consisting of a photocell that converts light to an electric current. The cell is connected to a moving coil meter that indicates the current as lux. The most suitable type for workplace measurements should have a range of 0–2500 lux and should have the photocell separate from the meter, but connected via a length of cable. This arrangement allows the meter to be read without the observer overshadowing the cell. The photocell should be corrected to take into account the effects of light falling upon it from an oblique angle (cosine-corrected) and preferably colour-corrected to allow measurements to be taken over a wide range of lamps and with daylight. Manufacturers of these meters do provide colour-correction charts for use with instruments, which approximate the illuminance. Typical colour-correction factors are given in Table 6.1. The accuracy of photometers should be checked from time to time using sources of known intensity. Examples of such instruments are shown in Figs 6.1 and 6.2.

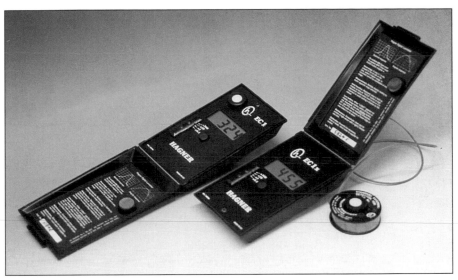

Fig. 6.1. Photoelectric photometer (Hagner Photometric Instruments Ltd).

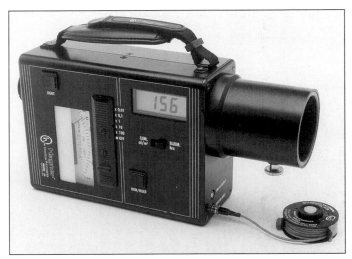

Fig. 6.2. Hagner Universal Photometer (Hagner Photometric Instruments Ltd).

Hagner Universal Photometer

This is an instrument for measuring luminance or the brightness of light given off or reflected from a surface. It consists of a photoelectric cell coupled to a meter calibrated in candela m^{-2}.

There is a viewfinder similar to a camera through which the surface to be measured is observed and the cell only responds to the light emitted from the surface contained within the field of the viewfinder. Thus to make a measurement the instrument has to be held up to the eye and pointed at the surface being tested as shown in Fig. 6.2.

Table 6.1. Colour correction factors of a typical photometer

Light source	Multiply reading by
Fluorescent:	
warm white	1.27
daylight	1.20
colour matching	1.05
natural	1.14
Sodium low power	1.30
Sodium	1.19
Mercury vapour	1.26

Daylight factor meter

These instruments normally consist of a selenium barrier-layer photocell cosine-corrected by means of a filter that compensates for light reflected from the detecting cell surface above it and connected by way of sensitivity control to a micro-ammeter. A hinged louvred mask closes over the cell for outdoor use, which reduces the overall illumination of the photocell and admits light only from an elevation of 40–50°, that is from that zone of the sky where the brightness is numerically equal to the illuminance of the whole sky. Indoor readings are taken with the mask hinged clear of the photocell for increased sensitivity with a non-directional characteristic. An instrument of this type is illustrated in Fig. 6.3.

To measure the daylight factors in a room

Aim

Many workplaces rely upon daylight for the majority of the day's illumination, artificial light being provided only when the worker considers it is too dark to see properly. There is often a tendency for the person to delay turning on the lights until the illumination has reached such a low level that the work is affected or a higher than normal risk of an accident occurring is present. Therefore, it is normal to provide some supplementary artificial lighting to boost the daylight entering through the windows that may be operating all of the time or switched on under the influence of a light sensor.

Some scheme or programme of illumination control may have to be calculated based upon the measurement of daylight factors. An opinion on daylight factors expressed by Smith (1995) states as follows:

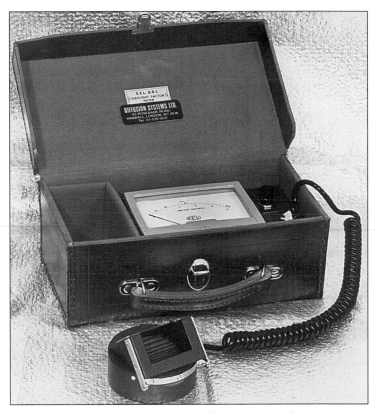

Fig. 6.3. EEL daylight factor meter (Diffusion Systems Ltd).

It is generally accepted that when the average daylight factor is greater than typically 5%, the building interior will give the appearance of being lit cheerfully by daylight. Conversely, if the average daylight factor drops below typically 2%, natural daylight will rarely be satisfactory and artificial lighting is likely to be required constantly.

Smith 1990

Also, the amount of daylight reaching a workplace may change due to the presence of external changes affecting the amount of light falling upon a window for such reasons as the erection of a new building or item of industrial plant. There may also be the need to check for excessive daylight causing glare on some workplace for which the remedy is shading or screening using such items as venetian blinds but which may affect the daylight illumination on some other part of the room. For these and other reasons it is useful to be able to check the amount of natural daylight falling upon a workplace.

Equipment required
A daylight factor meter or a lightmeter (see below) graph paper, a tape measure.

Method
Measure the room size and sketch a plan of it on the graph paper, noting the positions of workplaces and items of equipment. The windows should be measured for effective area and those values marked on the sketch at the appropriate positions.
1   Close the louvred mask over the photocell of the meter.
2   Stand outside or by an open window and hold the instrument at a convenient height to read the scale, direct the louvres towards an unobstructed area of overcast sky. Note that daylight factors can only be measured under an overcast sky.
3   Adjust the sensitivity control so that the meter scale reads X1 to X2, that is, line up the meter needle with the line indicating X1 or X2.
4   Return to the room to be measured and switch off all artificial lighting. Swing the louvred mask completely clear of the photocell (i.e. open) and, taking care not to obstruct the daylight, hold the meter at various positions in the room and note the reading. It is advisable to move away from the window in increments of 0.5 m, noting the results as laid out in the result sheet in Table 6.2. The meter will read directly in terms of percentage daylight. It may be necessary to alter the sensitivity of the meter.
5   Repeat this for various traverses across the room so that the whole area is covered. It is suggested that the traverses be 1 m apart.

Unfortunately, daylight factor meters are hard to find and do not appear to be made now (1998). However, a daylight factor survey can still be made using a normal lux meter by measuring and noting the level of illumination outside the room window on a cloudy day and immediately returning to the room. The survey can be undertaken from step 4 above, recording the lux readings instead of the daylight factor. The internal readings divided by the outside illumination value expressed as a percentage will give the daylight factors.

Results
Transfer the results to the sketch and draw contours through points of equal daylight as shown in Fig. 6.4.

Table 6.2. Suggested results sheet for daylight factors

Distance from window wall (m)	Daylight factors in traverse									
	1	2	3	4	5	6	7	8	9	....
0.5										
1.0										
1.5										
2.0										
2.5										
3.0										

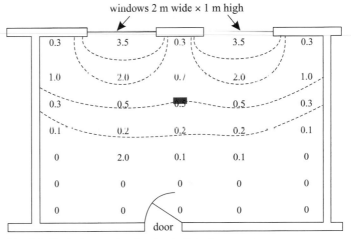

windows 2 m wide × 1 m high

0.3	3.5	0.3	3.5	0.3
1.0	2.0	0.7	2.0	1.0
0.3	0.5	0.5	0.5	0.3
0.1	0.2	0.2	0.2	0.1
0	2.0	0.1	0.1	0
0	0	0	0	0
0	0	0	0	0

door

Fig. 6.4. Typical room plan showing daylight factors and contours.

To undertake a lighting survey of a workroom

Aim
In order to fully understand the distribution of light in a room and to determine whether workplace illumination levels are suitable and sufficient for the work to be undertaken, two stages of assessment are required. The first is to complete a subjective examination of the general illumination and the second is to follow that up with some organised measurement of lighting levels.

Equipment required
A portable photoelectric photometer, a visual assessment form, plain and graph paper, tape measure, pencils and, if possible, a camera.

Method

Preliminaries

1   Draw a sketch plan of the room to show the principal working surfaces, windows, light fittings and other relevant features. This should be done to scale if possible. It may be necessary to draw separate floor and ceiling plans to avoid confusion between the furniture and the light fittings. These can be done on tracing paper or translucent sheets so that one can overlay the other. In order to assist the memory, section drawings can be made through windows to show their dimensions and the positions of light fittings, or an 'exploded' sketch can be made giving the same information. It is also useful to take a photograph of the room from various positions, but failing that an isometric sketch can be made on which wall colours and the nature of surfaces can be noted.

2   Measure the major dimensions of the room and note them on the sketch plans. Note and record also the nature of the lighting in use, whether it is daylight or artificial or a mixture of both, and record the type of lamp, its wattage and the type of diffuser or holder in use. The state of the room should be noted with regard to cleanliness, that is, observe whether the light fittings, lamps and windows are clean or dirty and the reflectances of the principal room surfaces.

Visual assessment

Having spent some minutes in the room it is useful to make a visual assessment. Identify any specific aspects of the lighting installation that should be examined in detail. Decide if illuminance on working surfaces appears to be satisfactory and, if not, determine the reason why and in which parts of the room. Ascertain whether the present use of the space differs from the original purpose for which the lighting was designed and determine what the illuminance levels and the daylight factors should be for such a purpose-built room from codes of practice such as the CIBSE Code (see Further reading).

Determine whether there are any undesirable shadows or reflections on the work. Notice whether the lighting fittings or windows cause discomfort or disability glare when seen separately or together and observe whether the windows are obstructed by internal furnishings or equipment and by outside trees, walls or other buildings, which may affect the illumination.

If the nature of the work requires the recognition of different colours, note whether the colour rendering of the lights is satisfactory. This may have to be done by removing some of the coloured material to the window or outside to observe it under natural daylight to see whether the colour changes.

Notice whether there is any flicker from discharge lamps including fluorescent tubes and if any stroboscopic effects on moving machinery are present (rotating items may appear stationary if running at the same speed as the mains frequency).

The following check list may be helpful to undertake this subjective visual assessment:

1   Adequacy of lighting.
2   Suitability of lighting to function of room.
3   Shadows on work surfaces.
4   Reflections affecting work stations.
5   Glare from windows and lights:
      (a) causing discomfort; and
      (b) causing disability.
6   Obstructions to windows from inside or outside.
7   Colour rendering.
8   Cleanliness of light fittings, windows and wall surfaces.
9   Flicker.
10 Distribution of light over the whole room.
11 General impressions of whether satisfactory or not.

It is useful to chat to the people occupying the room to establish their subjective feelings about the lighting levels and whether any discomfort is experienced. They may also be in a position to suggest where improvements might be made.

Measurement

If the weather conditions are correct, that is, with an overcast sky, the measurement of illumination levels can be preceded by a daylight factor survey as shown previously. This will show the distribution of daylight, the minimum daylight factor and the values at specific work positions.

Using the photoelectric photometer measure the illuminance readings at all work stations and on every work surface. This should be done with the normal workplace lighting switched on, that is, with general and local lamps on. In addition to this an imaginary grid of 1 m squares should be drawn up and illuminance readings taken in the centre of each grid square with both general lighting only on and with general and local lighting on. Guidance is required on what the minimum number of measuring points should be, and this can be done by determining a room index, RI, calculated from the equation given below and Table 6.3.

$$RI = \frac{L \times W}{H_m (L + W)}$$

Table 6.3. The relationship between room index RI and minimum number of measuring points

Room index	Minimum number of measuring points
0	4
0.9	9
1.9	16
2.0	25
3.0	36
3.4	36
5.1	36

where: L is room length

W is room width

H_m is mounting height above the working plane (vertical height of lamp above floor minus height of working surface)

Example: A room 10 m long × 5 m wide has flush mounted luminaires 2.5 m above floor; desk heights are 0.85 m above floor. Calculate the RI and determine the minimum number of measuring positions for a lighting survey.

$$L = 10 \text{ m}, \ W = 5 \text{ m}, \ H_m = 2.5 - 0.85 = 1.65 \text{ m}$$

$$RI = \frac{10 \times 5}{1.65 \, (10 + 5)} = 2.02$$

From Table 6.3, the minimum number of measuring positions is 25. Measurements should be taken in a horizontal plane, ideally at 0.85 m above floor level. Measuring points within 0.5 m of the boundary walls are not appropriate.

To use the photometer

1 With the cell disconnected adjust the zero as instructed.

2 Connect the cell to the meter.

3 If the cell is separate from the meter and connected by a cable, lay the cell on the surface to be measured and by standing as far from it as possible, so as not to overshadow it, read the meter by starting at the highest range setting and reducing the range step by step until the indicator gives an adequate deflection.

4 Correct the readings in accordance with the manufacturer's correction code and note the results directly on the plan.

If luminance readings are required of the floor, walls, ceilings and work surfaces then the Universal Photometer should be used as follows:

1   Remove from case and check the meter's mechanical zero and adjust if necessary.

2   Check the battery charge condition as indicated by the maker's instructions. This normally involves turning the range finder to any range and depressing a battery check button. If the pointer swings beyond a set mark the battery is in good condition but if the swing is insufficient replace the battery with a good one. Do not attempt to take readings with a low battery as the readings will be meaningless.

3   Hold the meter up to the eye and point it at the surface to be measured by viewing through the viewfinder. The surface being measured is that seen within the target circle.

4   Move the control switch to 'Lum. Internal Cell' and turn the meter range switch step by step until an adequate deflection is obtained on the meter. The actual value of luminance is obtained by multiplying the meter reading by the range value used.

5   Note the results.

Results and calculations

If further calculations are required in addition to recording the results on the plans then they should be tabulated as shown in Tables 6.4, 6.5 and 6.6.

Table 6.4. Recording of illuminance results

Measuring position (as shown in sketch)	Illuminance E (lux)	
	With general light only	With general and local light
Total		
Mean		

Calculate the diversity factor from:

$$DF = \frac{\text{minimum illuminance}}{\text{mean illuminance}}$$

Calculate the utilisation factor from:

Table 6.5. Recording of luminance and reflectance results

Surface	Luminance (Cd m^{-2})	Reflectance $= \dfrac{\text{luminance}}{\text{mean illuminance}}$
Floor		
Walls: 1		
Walls: 2		
Walls: 3		
Walls: 4		
Ceiling		
Horizontal machine surfaces: 1		
Horizontal machine surfaces: 2		
Horizontal machine surfaces: 3		
Horizontal machine surfaces: etc.		
Vertical machine surfaces: 1		
Horizontal machine surfaces: 2		
Horizontal machine surfaces: 3		
Horizontal machine surfaces: etc.		

Table 6.6. Basic room data sheet

Date and time of survey	
Place surveyed (address)	
Room surveyed	
Purpose of survey	
Principle visual tasks	
Planes on which work is done	
Recommended CIBSE Code values: illuminance daylight factor	
Dimensions of room: length width height	
Windows: width height	

Comments on nature of lighting	
Daylight: side windows roof glazing	
Artificial light	
Daylight and artificial	
State of fittings: clean/dirty	
State of floors: clean/dirty	
State of windows: clean/dirty	
State of walls: clean/dirty	
State of diffusers: clean/dirty	
State of mountings: clean/dirty	
Lamp/luminaire: types wattage	

$$UF = \frac{\text{mean illuminance with artificial light} \times \text{area of room}}{\text{total wattage of lamps in room}}$$

Calculate the maintenance factor from:

$$MF = \frac{\text{mean illuminance} \times \text{floor area}}{UF \times \text{total wattage of lamps}}$$

Record luminance in candela m^{-2} on a table similar to Table 6.5 and calculate reflectance on the same table. Record basic room data on a table similar to Table 6.6.

By comparing the results with the standards of workplace illumination recommended in the CIBSE Code, places that require attention can be listed. Improvements can involve either a general cleaning and redecoration of the area or a redesign of the lighting system.

To measure glare at a display screen workstation using a Hagner photometer

Background

The European Community Council Directive 90/270/EEC lays down minimum safety and health requirements for work with display screens. Member countries have written their own regulations based on that directive, and in the UK the Health and Safety (Display Screen Equipment) Regulations came into force on 1 January 1992. One of the requirements of the Directive is to ensure that the screen is free from reflective glare and reflections liable to to cause discomfort. The brightness and contrast of the characters on the screen must also be easily adjustable. in addition, there is a duty on employers to make an analysis of the workstation in order to evaluate the safety and health conditions which might give rise to possible risks to eyesight, physical problems and problems of mental stress.

Unsatisfactory lighting of the screen, the immediate surroundings and the far field may give rise to discomfort leading to one of the problems listed above. Discomfort glare can occur when the immediate background to the screen is too brightly lit, for example if the screen is in front of a window during daylight hours. Also, this type of glare can be caused in older open-plan or large offices where light fittings are not recessed into the ceiling; successive rows of lights can merge into a large illuminated mass. If such a source of light is seen just above the screen glare is experienced. Using the Hagner photometer it is possible to measure the light output of the screen, the immediate surroundings and the far field.

Equipment required
A Hagner photometer, small screwdriver

Method

Zeroing and calibration

1 Switch instrument on to × 10 000 scale.
2 Check battery on photometer; replace as necessary.
3 Check the zero by darkening the internal cell by pressing the appropriately labelled button just above the meter, turning the scale switch to × 1 and adjust zero by turning the screw labelled SET ZERO. Turn the scale to × 10 000 before releasing the DARKEN INTERNAL CELL button.
4 Calibrate by directing the photometer to towards a surface of known illuminance and, if the meter fails to give the correct reading, remove the plug labelled L and adjust the screw with a small screwdriver until it does, then replace the plug.
5 The instrument is now ready for use.

Use

6 Sit in the operator's chair, observe the screen and note any reflections from surrounding light sources such as luminaires or windows.
7 Adjust the angle of the screen to eliminate these.
8 If these cannot be eliminated move the orientation of the whole work station until they are.
9 Raise the Hagner photometer to the eye, point it to the screen and fill the viewfinder with light from the screen.
10 Observe the reading in the viewfinder scale.
Note: it may be necessary to adjust the scale switch to obtain a readable value. A typical desktop computer screen with dark letters on a bright background should emit light at a value of between 20 and 30 $Cd\ m^{-2}$, but a laptop computer with white letters on a dark background will emit only 3–7 $Cd\ m^{-2}$.
11 Still keeping the instrument to one's eye, move the viewfinder to the side of the screen so that it is receiving light from the immediate background and note the reading.
Note: this may be from office furniture, carpet or curtains whose value may vary from 2 to 8 $Cd\ m^{-2}$, but it may be from a window whose value could be 150–2000 $Cd\ m^{-2}$ or merged light fittings, which also could be over 1000 $Cd\ m^{-2}$.
12 Repeat for the other side and the top and note the highest value.
13 Move the viewfinder to a wider background and repeat.

Results and calculations

Take the screen reading as 100% and express the other readings as a percentage of the screen. The ideal result should show the screen at 100%, the immediate background as 30% and the wider background as 10%, i.e. a ratio of 100 : 30 : 10

Example 1: Screen of a desktop computer 25 Cd m^{-2}, immediate background (office furniture) 7 Cd m^{-2}, far background (end wall of office) 2.5 Cd m^{-2}.

Screen $\dfrac{25}{25} \times 100\% = 100\%$,

Immediate background $\dfrac{7}{25} \times 100\% = 28\%$,

Far background $\dfrac{2.5}{25} \times 100\% = 10\%$

Ratio of results: 100 : 28 : 10.
Result: satisfactory situation – no discomfort glare.

Example 2: Screen of a desktop computer 25 Cd m^{-2}, immediate background (other buildings through window) 26 Cd m^{-2}, far background (window, grey sky) 200 Cd m^{-2}.

Screen $\dfrac{25}{25} \times 100\% = 100\%$,

Immediate background $\dfrac{26}{25} \times 100\% = 104\%$,

Far background $\dfrac{200}{25} \times 100\% = 800\%$

Ratio of results: 100 : 104 : 800.
Result: very unsatisfactory situation – discomfort glare very likely.

Further reading

The Chartered Institute of Building Services Engineers (1985) *The CIBSE Code for Interior Lighting*. CIBSE, London. (For address see Appendix II.)

European Council Directive 1990 90/270/EEC on the minimum safety and health requirements for work with display screen equipment, OJ No. L 156/14, Brussels.

Longmore, J. (1980) Light. In: *Occupational Hygiene* (eds H.A. Waldron & J.M. Harrington), pp. 195–224. Blackwell Scientific Publications, Oxford.

SI (1993) Guidance on Regulations. *Health and Safety (Display Screen Equipment) Regulations 1992*. HSE Books, Sudbury, Suffolk.

Smith, N.A. (1991) *Lighting for Occupational Hygienists*. HHSC Handbook No. 7. H&H Scientific Consultants Ltd, Leeds.

Smith, N.A. (1995) Light and lighting. In: *Occupational Hygiene* (eds H.A. Waldron & J.M. Harrington), pp. 167–190. Blackwell Science, Oxford.

7 Radiation

Introduction

Radiation is a hazard that can occur in the workplace but is sufficiently specialised to remain outside the jurisdiction of most health and safety personnel unless they have undergone special training for its measurement and control. When it occurs in a workplace it is normally an integral part of the work process and is present with the full knowledge of all concerned, having the necessary safeguards built in. Unlike dust, gases or heat, a radiation hazard cannot be immediately perceived by the normal human senses; therefore no warning signs are noticed nor can avoiding action be taken. Because of its specialised nature, the reader is strongly advised to consult an expert whenever a problem is suspected or further information is required. In the UK, under the Ionising Radiation Regulations, 1985, a Radiation Protection Advisor (RPA) needs to be appointed for certain conditions.

There are two types of radiation: ionising and non-ionising. Examples encountered in work areas are given in Table 7.1 and the frequencies and wavelengths of the various forms of electromagnetic radiation are shown in Fig. 7.1.

Table 7.1. Examples of ionising and non-ionising radiation

Ionising radiation	Non-ionising radiation
Alpha (α)	Radiowaves
Beta (β)	Microwaves
Gamma (γ)	Visible light (e.g. lasers)
X-rays (Roentgen rays)	and/or infrared
Neutrons	Ultraviolet

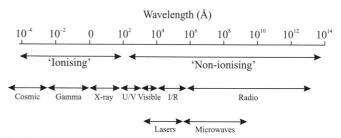

Fig. 7.1. Electromagnetic spectrum.

Ionising radiation

Ionising radiation is produced during radioactive decay, which on interaction with body tissue loses energy. This type of radiation can be hazardous to health because, if it penetrates living tissue, the resulting ionisation can cause chemical changes in the body that lead to harmful effects.

The damage caused by radiation exposure can result in two types of effects:

1 *Non-stochastic* (for example, cataract of eye lens, skin ulceration and impaired fertility), which are assumed to vary in severity with the level of radiation dose received, but are not detectable until a threshold dose has been received.

2 *Stochastic* (for example, induction of carcinogenesis and genetic damage), which are such that the risk increases progressively with the dose received. There is no detectable threshold. It is assumed that the severity of a stochastic effect, if it occurs at all, is independent of the level of dose responsible for it.

The hazard from radiation can arise either from the uniform irradiation of the whole body or part of a body (external radiation) or from irradiation due to ingested, inhaled or absorbed radioactive material concentrating in particular organs and tissues of the body (internal radiation).

Background radiation

Artificial ionising radiation has been used for several decades in the development and understanding of the sciences including medicine, and in industry. Naturally occurring radioactivity, on the other hand, has always existed and pervades the whole environment. Thus background radiation varies from place to place and is made up of radiation from the sun and outer space, from naturally occurring radioactive materials on earth, and radioactive aerosols and gases in the atmosphere and can amount to 200 μSv per year. Added to this, recently, are artificial sources of radiation such as escape from nuclear installations, fall-out from nuclear explosions, radioactive waste and occupational exposure. Natural and artificial radiations are the same in kind and effect.

In common with other hazards encountered in work environments, radiation carries a risk of causing harm and employees must be protected from unnecessary or excessive exposure to it. Although radiation of natural origin causes the highest exposure, much of it is unavoidable – although some control could be effected. Exposure to artificial radiation is more readily controlled by a system of radiological protection procedures. Some of these aspects will be mentioned briefly later in this chapter.

Basic concepts and quantities

All matter is composed of *elements*. Elements consist of character-istic *atoms*, which contain a relatively small *nucleus*, and a number of *electrons*, which are negatively charged particles with a small mass that may be imagined encircling the nucleus within *shells* with indefinite boundaries. The nucleus contains *protons*, which are larger than the electrons in mass and carry a positive charge, and *neutrons*, which are also large in mass but carry no electric charge. When the number of protons equal the number of electrons the atom is electrically neutral or stable.

The number of protons in an atom is called the *atomic number* and is represented by the symbol Z. The number of protons deter-mines the chemical properties of the atom and so defines the elements. The elements are listed in the *periodic table* in ascending order of the atomic number. For example, the first six elements are shown in Table 7.2.

Table 7.2. The first six elements of the periodic table

Element	No. of protons
Hydrogen (H)	1
Helium (He)	2
Lithium (Li)	3
Beryllium (Be)	4
Boron (B)	5
Carbon (C)	6

The *mass* of an atom is fixed and is the number of protons plus neutrons. The very small mass of the electrons is ignored. The *mass number* is the number of protons plus number of neutrons and is represented by A. For example, in the case of hydrogen:

Number of protons	$= 1$
Number of neutrons	$= 0$
Number of electrons (ignore mass)	$\underline{= 1}$
Therefore, the mass number (A)	$= 1$

The complete classification of any element is as follows:

$$_Z^A X_N$$

where X is the chemical symbol of element, N, the number of neutrons and protons (nucleus), A, the mass number, and Z, the atomic number (or number of protons).

For hydrogen the classification is:

$_1^1 H_0$	$_1^2 H_1$	$_1^3 H_2$
hydrogen	deuterium	tritium

Usually the chemical symbol of the element is written with the mass number only since the atomic number is always the same. For example:

^{14}C or carbon-14 for $^{14}_{6}C$.

It can be seen that although all the atoms of a particular element, in this case hydrogen, contain the same number of protons, they may occur with different numbers of neutrons. This means that an element can have several types of atoms. These different forms are called *isotopes* or *nuclides* of the element. The isotopes for helium ($Z = 2$) are ^{3}He, ^{4}He and ^{5}He or helium-3, helium-4 and helium-5 respectively. Note that all the isotopes of a given element are chemically identical, since the chemical properties are determined by the atomic number of the element.

Some atoms are unstable. The stability of a nucleus is determined by the numbers of neutrons and protons, their configuration and the forces they exert on each other. To attain stability, changes take place within the atom that result in the emission of radiation. The process of spontaneous transformation of an unstable atom into an atom of another element while emitting radiation is called *radioactivity* (Fig. 7.2).

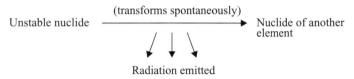

Fig. 7.2. Decay of an unstable nuclide to a stable one.

An atom whose nucleus is unstable is known as a *radioactive isotope* or *radionuclide*. The transformation is termed *decay* and the emission of radiation is called *ionising radiation*. For example, carbon-14 is a radionuclide that decays by emitting β radiation to nitrogen-14, a stable nuclide (Fig. 7.3).

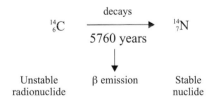

Fig. 7.3. Decay of Carbon 14.

Radioactivity decay can take place in stages, the last decay product being a stable isotope (Fig. 7.4).

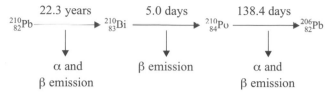

Fig. 7.4. An example of decay in stages: lead to bismuth to polonium to lead, with half-lives of intermediate products.

Of the 1700 or so known nuclides about 280 are stable. The behaviour of stable and unstable nuclei and the characteristic of any nucleus can be found in a *nuclide chart.*

Types of radiation

The main forms of radiation that result from radioactive decay are either particulate (α and β particles) or electromagnetic (γ rays and X-rays).

Alpha (α) *particles* are streams of positively charged helium nuclei, which are comprised of two protons plus two neutrons. The particles are heavy and their range in air is 2–5 cm. They are easily stopped by paper, thin foil or the skin. Their range in body tissue is less than 1 mm and they are only hazardous if α-emitting materials are taken into the body. Examples of application of α sources are in static eliminators, smoke detectors and thickness gauges.

Beta (β) particles have mass and charge equal to an electron. Beta rays are streams of negatively charged particles or electrons. Their range in air is 4–5 m and they can be stopped by thin layers of water, glass, perspex or aluminium. Their range of penetration depends on their energy. They have greater penetrating power in body tissue, approximately 2 cm, and β emitters are also hazardous if taken into the body. Examples of applications of β-emitting sources are in static eliminators, direct and back-scattered thickness gauges, luminescent materials and selected radioactive materials used in research and diagnostics.

Gamma (γ) *rays* are discrete quantities of energy without mass or charge and are propagated as waves. Gamma rays are electromagnetic radiations similar to light and radiowaves but with shorter wavelengths and higher energies. Their range in air can be greater than 100 m and they are highly penetrating to body tissue and are hazardous when external to the body. They can be attenuated by heavy shielding materials such as lead and concrete. Gamma radiation is used in medical diagnosis and therapy, thickness gauges, level gauges, and pipe line flow rate measurement. Gamma rays and X-rays are indistinguishable from each other and only differ in how they are produced.

Occupational exposure can also occur with two other forms of ionising radiation:

X-rays are also electromagnetic rays with approximately 60 m range in air. They are less penetrating to body tissue than γ rays but equally hazardous when external to the body. They too can be attenuated by high-density materials like lead or concrete. X-rays are used in radiography and fluoroscopy and are produced by bombarding a metal target with electrons in an evacuated tube.

Neutrons are electrically neutral particles. Their range in air is greater than 100 m and they are highly penetrating to body tissues. When neutrons are first produced in a reactor or in a particle accelerator such as a cyclotron, they are known as fast neutrons. Thick shields of materials containing light atoms such as water, wax or graphite are effective in slowing them. The slow neutrons can then be efficiently absorbed by shields of cadmium or boron. Neutron-emitting radioactive sources are used for activation analysis in a variety of medical and industrial applications, in prospecting for oil and gas, for measuring the moisture content of soils and cements and for testing reactor instrumentation.

Energy

The energy with which radiations are produced is expressed in *electron volts* (eV). This is equivalent to the energy gained by an electron in passing through a potential difference of 1 volt. Multiples of this unit are commonly used, mainly the kiloelectron volt (keV) and megaelectron volt (MeV).

$$1 \text{ keV} = 1000 \text{ eV}$$
$$1 \text{ MeV} = 1000 \text{ keV} = 1\,000\,000 \text{ eV}$$

Some radionuclides produce more than one type of energy. Examples are given in Table 7.3.

For non-β radiation, the electron volt is used as a unit energy from the relationship,

$$E_k = 0.5 \, mv^2,$$

where E_k = kinetic energy
m = mass of particle, and
v = velocity of particle.

Activity

A radioactive material does not emit radiation indefinitely. The activity or source strength of a radionuclide is the rate at which spontaneous decay occurs in it. As soon as a radionuclide is formed, its activity decays with time and this process cannot be changed.

Table 7.3. Example of types of radiation emitted by a selection of radionuclides (from Amersham Manual, 2nd edn)

Isotope	Half-life	Type of decay	Beta energies (MeV)	Gamma energies (MeV)	Specific γ-ray constant
Americium-241	458 (years)	α	5.44 (13%)	0.026 (2.5%)	
		α	5.48 (85%)	0.033 (weak)	
				0.060 (36%)	
Caesium-137	30 (years)	β^-	0.51 (95%)	0.662 (86%)	3.3
		β^-	1.17 (5%)		
Carbon-14	5760 (years)	β^-	0.159 (100%)		
Chromium-51	27.8 (days)	EC	(100%)	0.323 (9%)	0.16
				0.005 (X-rays)	
Hydrogen-3	12.26 (years)	β^-	0.018 (100%)		
Radon-22	3.825 (days)	α	5.48 (100%)		
Rhodium-106	30 (s)	β^-	1.5 (1%)	0.51 (20.5%)	1.7
		β^-	2.0 (2%)	0.62 (10.8% −	
		β^-	2.4 (11%)	others up to 2.9)	
		β^-	3.0 (8%)		
		β^-	3.5 (78%)		
Sodium-22	2.6 (years)	β^+	0.54 (90.5%)	0.51 (from β^+)	12.0
		β^+	1.83 (0.06%)	1.28 (100%)	
		EC	(9.5%)		
Technetium-99^m	6 (h)	IT	(100%)	0.002 (10%)	
		(100%)		0.140 (90.1%)	
				0.142 (0.04%)	
Vanadium-52	3.8 (min)	β^-	2.73 (100%)	1.45 (100%)	7.4

EC denotes orbital electron capture by the nucleus resulting in emission of X-rays characteristic of the daughter element. Gamma rays can also be emitted.
IT denotes isometric transition.
Beta and gamma particles emit energy at different energy levels, which may vary.

The rate of decay depends on the type of radioactive substance. Activity is expressed in Becquerels (Bq) or disintegrations per second in SI units and was known as Curies (Ci) in Imperial Units. Multiples are frequently used, since:

$$1 \text{ Ci} = 37\ 000\ 000\ 000 \text{ Bq} = 37 \times 10^9 \text{ Bq}.$$

Table 7.4 gives the relationships between Becquerels and Curies.

Table 7.4. Relationships between Becquerels and Curies

1 becquerel (Bq)	$= 1 \text{ ds}^{-1}$ (2.7×10^{-11} Ci)
1 kilobecquerel (kBq)	$= 10^3 \text{ ds}^{-1}$ (2.7×10^{-8} Ci)
1 megabecquerel (MBq)	$= 10^6 \text{ ds}^{-1}$ (27 μCi)
1 gigabecquerel (GBq)	$= 10^9 \text{ ds}^{-1}$ (27 mCi)
1 terabecquerel (TBq)	$= 10^{12} \text{ ds}^{-1}$ (27 Ci)
1 picocurie	$= 3.7 \times 10^{-2} \text{ ds}^{-1}$
1 nanocurie	$= 3.7 \times 10^{1} \text{ ds}^{-1}$
1 microcurie	$= 3.7 \times 10^{4} \text{ ds}^{-1}$ ($= 37$ kBq)
1 millicurie	$= 3.7 \times 10^{7} \text{ ds}^{-1}$ ($= 37$ MBq)
1 curie	$= 3.7 \times 10^{10} \text{ ds}^{-1}$ ($= 37$ GBq)

The time taken for a radionuclide to decay to half of its original value is known as the *half-life*. Each radioactive substance has a unique and unalterable half-life. Half-lives range from millions of years to fractions of seconds. In successive half-lives, the activity of a radionuclide is reduced by decay to one-half, one-quarter, one-eighth, one-sixteenth and so on of the initial value. It is therefore possible to predict the activity remaining at any time. A stable nuclide is a radionuclide with an infinite half-life. Some examples of half-lives are given in Tables 7.3 and 7.5.

Table 7.5.   Half-lives of some nuclides

Nuclide	Half-life
Carbon-14	5760 (years)
Cobalt-60	5 (years)
Iodine-125	60 (days)
Phosphorus-32	14 (days)
Technetium-99^{m}	6 (hours)

To determine the activity of a sample

Aim
The aim is to determine the activity of a sample. It is necessary to know the strength of a source for various reasons. Many sophisticated techniques are available to determine this precisely, but the following is a simple technique to get some idea of the strength of a radioactive source.

Equipment required
A Mini assay type 6.20 counter or scaler rate meter type 6.9 (Fig. 7.5), a sample in sealed tube to fit into the well of the counter (Fig. 7.6), long-handled tongs, check source.

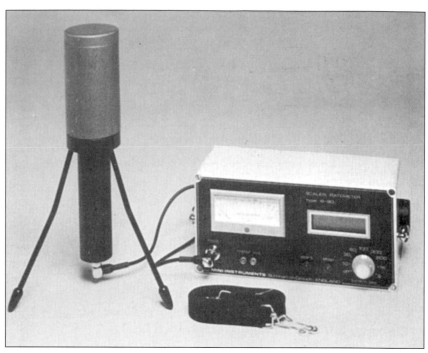

Fig. 7.5.   Scaler rate meter type 6.9 (Mini Instruments Ltd).

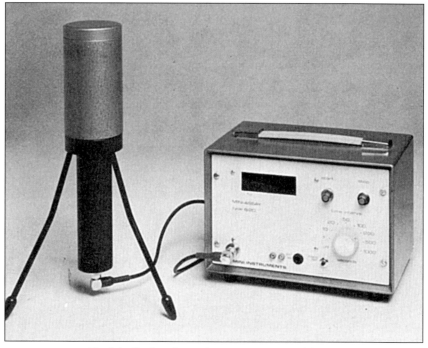

Fig. 7.6.   Single well crystal counter type 6.20 (Mini Instruments Ltd).

Method

1   Wear appropriate protective clothing and personal dosimeter.
2   Switch on the counter or rate meter and allow a few seconds for the needle display to settle.
3   Check that counter or rate meter is responding correctly with the check source.
4   Record the background count in disintegrations per second.
5   Using the tongs place the sample in the well. Record the count after it reaches a constant level in disintegrations per second.
6   Store sample in appropriate storage area.
7   Carry out calculation.

Calculations

Calculate the activity from the relationship:

$$\text{Efficiency (\%)} = \frac{\text{counts of samples (ds}^{-1}) - \text{background count (ds}^{-1})}{\text{activity (ds}^{-1})}$$

The efficiency of the counting system is the fraction of particles counted compared with the total number emitted. For example:

Counting efficiency $= 15\%$

Background count $= 60 \text{ ds}^{-1}$, and

Count of sample $= 555\ 060 \text{ ds}^{-1}$ (in a set period of time).

Rearranging the above relationship:

$$\text{Activity} = \frac{\text{sample count} - \text{background count}}{\text{efficiency}}$$

$$= \frac{555\ 060 - 60}{15}$$

$$= 37\ 000 \text{ ds}^{-1}$$

$$= 3.7 \times 10^4$$

$$= 37 \text{ kBq } (1\text{m Ci})$$

Possible problems

1   Although the check source indicates that the monitor is responding correctly, it needs to be inspected and calibrated annually by a competent person.
2   This technique is suitable only for the size of activity of a source used in laboratories.
3   This technique gives an approximate value only.

Radiation dose units

Exposure

When working with radioactive materials, exposure to the worker must be kept as low as reasonably achievable (ALARA). *Radiation exposure* is a quantity expressing the amount of ionisation caused in air by X or γ radiation. The unit *röntgen* (R) is equivalent to an exposure of 2.58×10^{-4} Coulombs per kilogramme (C kg^{-1}). Because the röntgen applies to X and γ radiation and their effect on air it is inadequate as a radiation exposure unit. The effect of radiation on human tissue is of interest. The energy deposition is often higher in tissue than in air so the concept of radiation absorbed dose (rad) was introduced.

Absorbed dose

Absorbed dose is a measure of energy deposition in any medium by all types of ionising radiation and expressed as the energy absorbed per unit mass of materials.

In the SI system of units, the unit of absorbed dose is called the *Gray* (Gy) and is defined as an energy deposition of one Joule per kilogram (1 J kg^{-1}).

The original unit of absorbed dose was the *rad* and was defined as energy deposition of 0.01 J kg^{-1}. Therefore,

1 Gy = 1 J kg^{-1} = 100 rad.

However, in biological systems the same absorbed dose of different types of radiation gives rise to different degrees of biological damage. To take this into account the absorbed dose of each type of radiation is multiplied by a *quality factor* (Q), which reflects the ability of the particular radiation to cause damage and is known as the *dose equivalent.*

Dose equivalent

In the SI system dose equivalent is the unit Sievert (Sv), which is related to the Gray as follows:

Dose equivalent (Sv) = absorbed dose Gy $\times Q \times N$,

where N is a further modifying factor, which accounts for other factors such as absorbed dose rate and fractionation.

The original unit for dose equivalent was the *rem*. Therefore,

Dose equivalent (rem) = absorbed dose (rad) $\times Q$.

N is normally assigned the value 1 and since 1 Gy = 100 rad it follows that 1 Sv = 100 rem.

The values of the quality factor depends on the density of ionisation caused by the radiation. They are given in Table 7.6.

Table 7.6. Types of radiation and quality factors

Types of radiation	Quality factors
X-rays, γ-rays and electrons	1
Thermal electrons	2.3
Fast neutrons and proton particles	10
α-particles	20

To calculate dose equivalent
An employee can be exposed to different types of radiation during a period of work. An indication of the exposure is required. For example, during an experiment an employee received the following amounts of radiation:

0.03 Gy (3 rad) γ dose
0.07 Gy (7 rad) X-ray dose
0.001 Gy (0.1 rad) fast neutron dose.

To calculate the total dose equivalent we use the relationship:

Dose equivalent = absorbed dose × quality factor.

Gamma dose equivalent   = 0.03 × 1   = 0.03 Sv (3 rem)

X-ray dose equivalent   = 0.07 × 1   = 0.07 Sv (7 rem)

Fast neutron dose equivalent = 0.001 × 10 = 0.01 Sv (1 rem)

Total dose equivalent   = 0.11 Sv (11 rem)

Dose rate
The dose rate is the rate at which a dose is received. The accumulation of dose received by an employee is equal to the dose rate multiplied by the time exposed to it. The shorter the time, the smaller the dose. The rate is usually expressed per hour. Therefore,

Total dose = dose rate × time,

where the dose rate is in Sieverts, and the time in hours.

But the Sievert is too large a unit for ordinary use, so millisieverts (mSv) and microsieverts (μSv) are used (see also Table 7.7):

1 mSv = 1/1000 Sv (100 mrem)
1 μSv = 1/1 000 000 Sv (0.1 mrem).

Table 7.7. Sub-multiples of exposure units

1 Gy = 1000 mGy = 1 000 000 µGy	
1 Sv = 1000 mSv = 1 000 000 µSv	
1 Sv = 100 rem	1 Gy = 100 rad
1 mSv = 100 mrem	1 mGy = 100 mrad
1 Sv = 0.1 mrem	1µGy = 0.1 mrad

To calculate dose
1   An employee is exposed to a uniform radiation of 5 µSv h^{-1} (0.5 mrem). What will be their dose in 3 hours?

Using the relationship:

Total dose = dose rate × time

and substituting

Total dose = 5 × 3

$$= 15 \text{ µSv (1.5 mrem).}$$

2   A classified worker is allowed to receive a dose equivalent of 1 mSv (100 mrem) in a week. How long can he work in an area in which the dose equivalent rate is 50 µSv h^{-1} (5 mrem h^{-1})?

Rearranging the relationship, we have

$$\text{Time} = \frac{\text{total dose}}{\text{dose rate}}$$

$$= \frac{1 \text{ mSv}}{50 \text{ µSv h}^{-1}}$$

$$= \frac{1000 \text{ µSv}}{50 \text{ µSv h}^{-1}}$$

$$= 20 \text{ h}$$

Dose limits

Safe dose limits are recommended by the International Commission on Radiation Protection (ICRP) and have been adopted in the UK by the HSE as published in the Ionising Radiation Regulations, 1985. The current dose limits for the UK are given in Table 7.8.

Table 7.8. Dose limits, which must not be exceeded in a calendar year

	Employees aged 18 years or over	Trainees aged under 18 years	Any other person
Whole body	50 mSv (5.0 rem)	15 mSv (1.5 rem)	5 mSv (0.5 rem)
Individual organs and tissues	500 mSv (50 rem)	150 mSv (15 rem)	50 mSv (5 rem)
Lens of the eye	150 mSv (50 rem)	45 mSv (4.5 rem)	15 mSv (1.5 rem)

Women of reproductive capacity:
Dose limit for the abdomen 13 mSv (1.3 rem) in any consecutive 3-month interval

Pregnant women:
Dose limit during the declared term of pregnancy 10 mSv (1.0 rem)

Derived limits

A derived limit (DL) is the limit for uniform external irradiation of the whole body. In the UK, for designated radiation employees, the dose limit is 50 mSv per year (see Table 7.8). The limit per hour can be calculated from:

Assuming the person works for 50 weeks the dose will be

$$\frac{50 \text{ mSv year}^{-1}}{50 \text{ weeks}}$$

$$= 1 \text{ mSv week}^{-1} \text{ (100 mrem week}^{-1})$$

$$= 1000 \text{ μSv week}^{-1}$$

Assuming a 40-hour week

$$\frac{1000 \text{ μSv week}^{-1}}{40 \text{h week}^{-1}}$$

$$= 25 \text{ μSv h}^{-1} \text{ (2.5 mrem h}^{-1})$$

The value of 25 μSv per hour is called a derived limit for irradiation of the whole body from external radiation.

Internal radiation is also controlled by limiting the airborne concentration and level of surface contamination. DLs for surface contamination can vary, depending on the type and toxicity of radioactive material and the classification of the area in which it can be handled safely.

Derived limits for air contamination that can be inhaled are often referred to as *derived air concentrations* (*DACs*) and these vary for the different radioactive substances.

The annual limits of intake (ALI) is the limit placed on the amount of a radionuclide ingested or inhaled in Becquerels, which would give a harm commitment to the organs it irradiates; the *committed dose equivalent* is equal to that resulting from whole body irradiation of 50 mSv (5 rem) in a year. These are estimated in ICRP 30 (an update of ICRP 2) and take into account chemical forms and translocation of radionuclides using three models; the models use the respiratory system, gastro-intestinal tract, and skeletal system. They relate the intake of radionuclides to organ dose and therefore to risk.

The derived air concentration is therefore the concentration that, breathed each week for 40 hours, leads to the absorption of ALI. ALI and DAC for selected radionuclides are listed in ICRP 30.

Procedures to minimise occupational dose

Occupational exposure comprises all dose equivalents and committed dose equivalents received at work. The nature and magnitude of occupational radiation exposure varies over a very wide range. Hence, the type and extent of individual monitoring required is dependent on the work environment. For example, a person working in a nuclear processing plant or in radioisotope manufacturing will require different levels of monitoring from someone working with low levels of radiation such as in tracer laboratories using unsealed radionuclides.

The Ionising Radiation Regulations, 1985, and the Recommendations of the ICRP control the handling, use and disposal of radioactive materials and apply to all premises where ionising radiations are handled.

To ensure control of exposure received, it is recommended that all persons using ionising radiation should register with a central body within an organisation so that the Health and Safety Services in that organisation are aware of the location and type of work being undertaken. All registered employees must undergo formal training in radiation protection principles and safe working procedures.

Dose limitation

Radiation dose limits are set so that non-stochastic effects are prevented completely and stochastic effects kept within acceptable limits. The principle of ALARA (as low as reasonably achievable) is encouraged. Employers are required to restrict the dose received by employees and other persons. This is achieved by (1) the use of engineering controls and design features, including shielding, containment of radioactive substances, ventilation, the provision of safety features and warning signs; (2) by administrative procedures, such as local rules; and (3) by designating categories to work areas (e.g. Controlled and Supervised) and personnel (e.g. Classified).

Where possible, work with unsealed sources should be carried out in fume cupboards behind appropriate shielding. In addition, safe systems of work in the form of site and departmental local rules covering procedures should be established. Facilities for personal hygiene, decontamination and waste disposal procedures and appropriate protective equipment should be provided. Compliance with these features should be monitored.

To ensure that the dose limits specified in the Regulations (see Table 7.8) are not exceeded, internal and external personal dosimetry is employed.

Regulation of work

Working areas are classified according to the potential level of exposure. These are:

Uncontrolled areas. The dose rate is less than 2.5 μSv h^{-1} so employees can spend all their working time here without exceeding 5 mSv per year.

Supervised areas. The dose rate does not exceed 7.5 μSv h^{-1} so employees should not exceed three-tenths of a dose limit (50 mSv year^{-1} $\approx$ 25 μSv h^{-1}; 25/3 $\approx$ 7.5 μSv h^{-1}), but the employees are subject to routine personal monitoring.

Controlled areas. The dose rate can exceed 7.5 μSv h^{-1} so employees are subject to medical surveillance and routine personal monitoring if they work regularly in these areas. Other employees can only enter it under a written system of work.

Restricted areas. The dose rate can exceed 25 μSv h^{-1} so access to these areas is subject to special precautions such as limitations of access time, the use of additional protective equipment and monitoring devices.

Dosimetry and medical surveillance

The UK Regulations require the monitoring of the doses received by Classified Persons and certain other employees and the maintenance of dose records (for 50 years) by a dosimetry service approved by the Health and Safety Executive.

On registration each worker is categorised for personal dosimetry based on the type and quantities of radioactive sources to be used and the nature of the work. If an employee is likely to exceed three-tenths of a set dose limit he or she is designated as a Classified Person and has to undergo more rigorous dosimetry and medical surveillance.

Film badges, body and extremity thermoluminescent (TLD) dosimeters can be used to monitor doses. These are supplied and analysed by an approved dosimetry service, such as the NRPB.

Dosimeters are usually changed every 4 weeks. Small pocket monitors, with pre-set alarms, are used for the daily monitoring of operators of large sealed sources or X-rays. Quarterly and annual doses are calculated and the records archived for the statutory period. Termination records are prepared by the approved dosimetry service when an employee leaves. A copy is given to the employer and another is forwarded to the HSE.

Medical surveillance of registered employees is carried out by an Approved Doctor (approved by the HSE). When an employer has an occupational health service, a medical officer is normally appointed as the Approved Doctor. Alternatively, the Employment Medical Advisory Service (EMAS) can be used to provide the health surveillance. The health record of Classified Persons, which must be kept for 50 years, is updated every 12 months, though a medical examination of the individual is not normally carried out unless personal dosimetry or other factors suggest that it would be advisable.

Control of radioactive substances

A system of accounting for all sources should be set up and administered by a central body within an organisation to ensure that the limits authorised for the site are not exceeded. A computer with appropriate software would simplify the collation of all acquisitions, stock levels, movements and disposals from monthly returns made by each user. These records are kept for 2 years and loss of radioactive material, above certain quantities defined in the Regulations, must be reported to the HSE. The accounting procedures required by the Radioactive Substances Act of 1960 and 1968 fulfils the requirements of the Ionising Radiations Regulations of 1985.

Monitoring of ionising radiation

Monitoring the levels of radiation in each 'Controlled' or 'Supervised' area is required, with records being kept for at least 2 years.

The local Rules should require that working areas and adjacent areas are monitored routinely. Hand-held monitors or wipe tests are normally carried out. More comprehensive monthly monitoring should be carried out in all working areas, with the emphasis placed on those most likely to be contaminated. All areas external to working areas (e.g. offices and corridors) should be monitored on a 3-monthly basis to ensure that contamination is not spreading.

All monitoring equipment must be tested and calibrated annually by a competent person (defined in the Regulations).

Assessment and notifications

Hazard assessment is an important requirement as it provides an opportunity to assess risks if work does not proceed according to plan. It is best carried out when a person seeks registration as a radiation worker, when new work is introduced and when major changes in existing work or facilities take place. Contingency plans for dealing with emergencies are developed and waste procedures defined and incorporated into the Local Rules.

Methods of protection

An external radiation hazard can arise from sources of radiation outside the body. It may be from a sealed or unsealed (sometimes called closed) source. A closed source is where the radioactive material is sealed in a strong container and cannot be removed by normal means; an unsealed source is a source such as a phial containing a liquid or powder; or it can arise from particles that are made to accelerate in machines and reactors. The hazard may be due to β, X, γ and neutron radiations. Alpha radiation is not normally regarded as an external hazard as α rays cannot penetrate the outer layers of skin.

There are four basic methods of protection against external radiation. These are shielding the worker from the radiation, arranging that the distance from the source to the worker is as long as possible, reducing the handling time to a minimum, and the restriction of the strength of the source to the minimum necessary for the task. A combination of these methods will give the protection necessary to ensure that doses are kept below the relevant dose limits in the work situation. It may be necessary to consult an expert to get the balance right. For example, it may be more dangerous if the source is shielded too much making its handling cumbersome and thereby increasing the exposure time.

Generally, shielding is the preferred method as it results in intrinsically safe working conditions. Reliance on distance or time of exposure involves continuous administrative control over employees. The different types of radiation have different powers of penetration but all of them can be stopped by some form of shielding materials. Advice may be obtained from manufacturers or a Radiation Protection Advisor (RPA) on the type and thickness of shielding necessary. The half-thickness or *half-value layer* (HVL) for a particular shielding material is the thickness required to reduce the intensity to one half of its incident value. Charts for various isotopes are available in the literature.

The intensity of a point source radiation decreases with increasing the distance, obeying the Inverse Square Law. Simply, this means that by doubling the distance the radiation level is reduced to one-quarter, by trebling the distance the radiation level is reduced to one-ninth, and so on. This works in reverse as well, that is, the intensity of radiation from a source increases with decreasing distance. Therefore, the nearer a worker is located to a source, the higher the radiation exposure. The radiation dose close to even a low activity source can be very high so it should never be touched with the bare hands; tongs or tweezers should always be used.

To demonstrate use of the Inverse Square Law

The dose rate from a source is 10 mSv h^{-1} at 100 cm. At what distance must an employee be placed to receive 40 mSv per hour?

The Inverse Square Law can be written as:

$$D_1 r_1^2 = D_2 r_2^2$$

where D_1 = the dose rate at distance r_1, and

D_2 = the dose rate at distance r_2 from the source.

Substituting

$$10 \times (100)^2 = 40 \times r_2^2$$

$$r_2^2 = \frac{10 \times (100)^2}{40}$$

$$\text{therefore } r_2 = \sqrt{\frac{10 \times 100 \times 100}{40}}$$

$$= 50 \text{ cm}$$

A useful expression for calculating the dose rate from a γ source is:

$$D = \frac{ME}{6r^2},$$

where D = dose rate in μSv h^{-1}

M = the activity of the source in MBq

E = the γ energy per disintegration of MeV, and

r = the distance from the source in metres.

Calculation of dose rate should always be confirmed with measurements of the dose rates using a dose rate monitor; an example is shown in Fig. 7.19.

Radiation monitoring

There are a plethora of radiation monitoring instruments on the market. Instruments that measure external radiation rely on detection devices based on the physical or chemical effects of radiation such as ionisation in gases, ionisation and excitation in certain solids, changes in chemical systems and activation of neutrons. They therefore vary in their sensitivity to radiation, the type of radiation to which they respond, their response to radiations of the same type but of different energies, the volume of the detector, the time taken to obtain a reading and the type of detector. Advice must be sought from an RPA on suitability and selection of appropriate instruments.

Radiation intensity is measured most commonly by an ionisation chamber, a proportional counter, Geiger–Muller counter

(a)

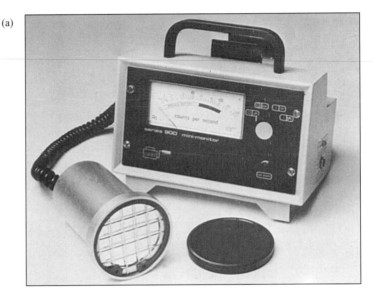

(b)

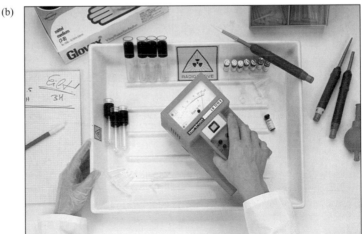

Fig. 7.7. (a) A 2-inch-diameter end window Geiger–Muller counter (Mini Instruments Ltd). (b) Ionising chamber (Berthold Instruments (UK) Ltd).

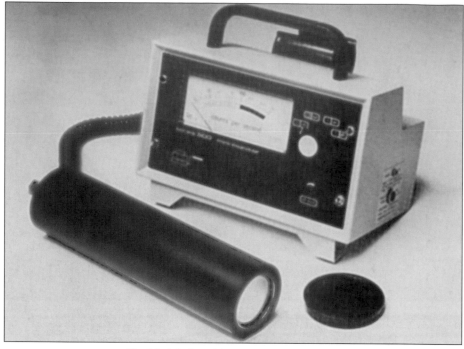

Fig. 7.8. Monitor with scintillation probe (Mini Instruments Ltd).

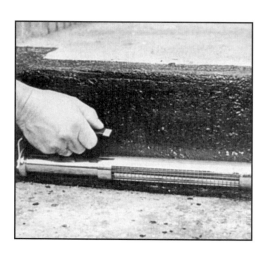

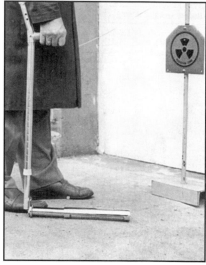

Fig. 7.9. Monitor with side window (Nuclear Enterprise Technology Ltd).

(Fig. 7.7) or a scintillation detector (Fig. 7.8). Most provide a numerical value known as a 'count' but to relate that count to true radiation intensity it is necessary to calibrate the instrument against a known value of intensity. The calibration factor can then be used to convert counts to other more useful units.

Monitors fall into three broad categories depending on the function they are required to perform:

1 Installed monitors, which are usually at fixed positions within radiation work areas and are used to monitor personal contamination (Fig. 7.15) or used to monitor the general radiation (Fig. 7.12b) and air contamination levels in the working environment.

2 Portable monitors, which are usually battery operated and can be carried from place to place as the need arises (Figs 7.7–7.11, 7,12a,c, 7.13 and 7.14). They are used for measurements during specific operations and for radiation and contamination surveys. A guide to the selection of the appropriate contamination monitor is given in Table 7.9. An example of a dose rate monitor is given in Fig. 7.19.

3 Personal monitors, which are worn by employees and which usually give instant dose received (Figs 7.16–7.18).

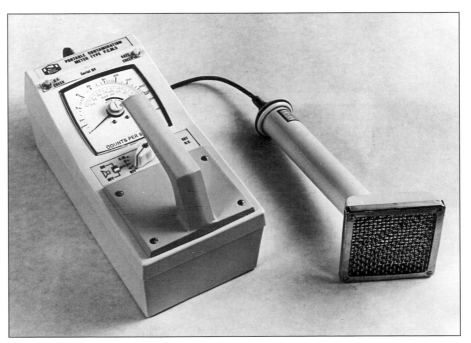

Fig. 7.10. Portable contamination meter (Nuclear Enterprise Technology Ltd).

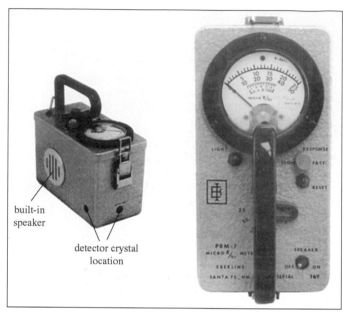

built-in
speaker

detector crystal
location

Fig. 7.11. Portable micro 'R' meter (Eberline Instruments Co. Ltd, now Southern Scientific).

Surface contamination monitoring

This is a convenient method of contamination monitoring. It is carried out to establish the presence of radiation contamination on surfaces such as workbench tops, clothing, skin. Direct measurements allow the contamination level to be calculated in MBq m^{-2} or they can be related to the derived working limits of surface contamination.

Table 7.9. Choice of contamination monitors (Mini Instruments Ltd)

Radionuclide	Contamination monitor
Tritium, nickel-63	No suitable detector — use swab
Carbon-14, sulphur-35, calcium-45	2-inch diameter end window, GM tube
Sodium-24, potassium-42, iron-59, cobalt-60, zinc-69, krypton-85, rubidium-106, silver-110, indium-114, tin-121, antimony-125	1-inch diameter end window, GM tube
Phosphorus-32, tin-90, potassium-42, cobalt-56	Side window, GM tube
Chromium-51, iron-55, cobalt-57, gallium-67, selenium-75	Scintillation probe, X-ray probe
Manganese-54, iodine-125	Scintillation probe
Technetium-99^{m}, chlorine-109	X-ray probe
Americium-241	γ-probe

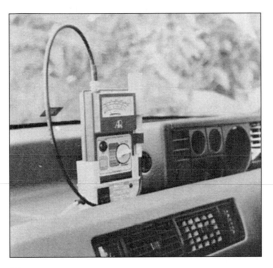

(a)

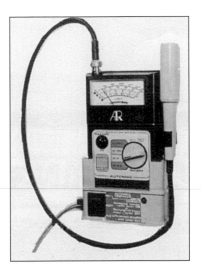

(b)

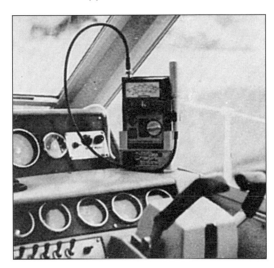

Fig. 7.12. Radiation measurement instrument (Radiation Components). (a) mobile; (b) fixed installation; (c) marine.

(c)

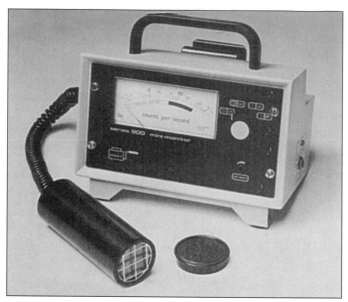

Fig. 7.13. 1-inch-diameter end window Geiger–Muller counter (Mini Instruments Ltd).

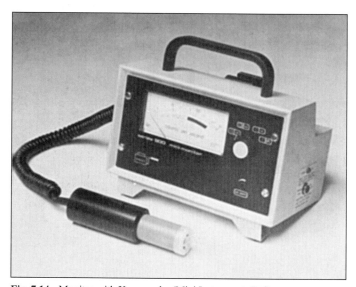

Fig. 7.14. Monitor with X-ray probe (Mini Instruments Ltd).

To carry out a contamination survey

Aim

To detect levels of contamination so that it can be removed before it spreads as it can not only ruin the work but pose both internal and external hazards to the employees. A survey can be carried out

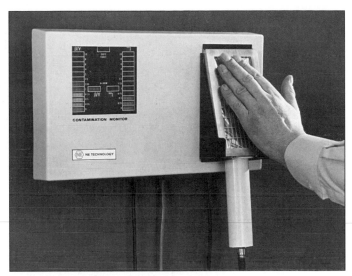

Fig. 7.15. An example of an installed monitor (Nuclear Enterprise Technology Ltd, now NE Technology).

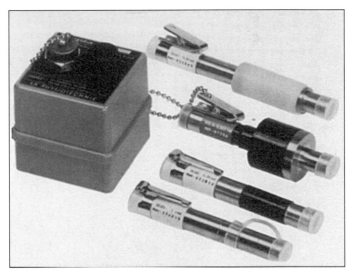

Fig. 7.16. Direct reading pocket dosimeter and charger (Eberline Instruments Co. Ltd, now Southern Scientific).

directly with a monitor if a suitable detector is available or by taking wipes of the surface to monitor the radiation indirectly. This method is known as a swab or smear survey.

Equipment required
Sketch plan of the work area, an appropriate portable contamination monitor.

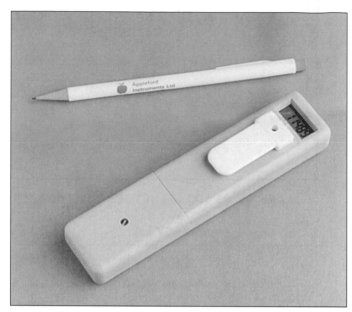

Fig. 7.17. Pocket dosimeter (Appleford Instruments Ltd).

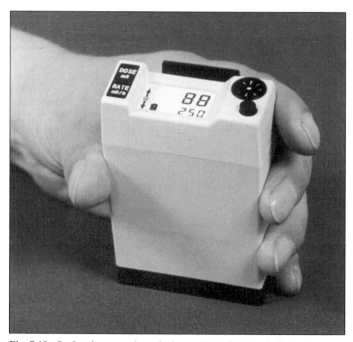

Fig. 7.18. Pocket dose rate alarm dosimeter (R.A. Stephen & Co. Ltd).

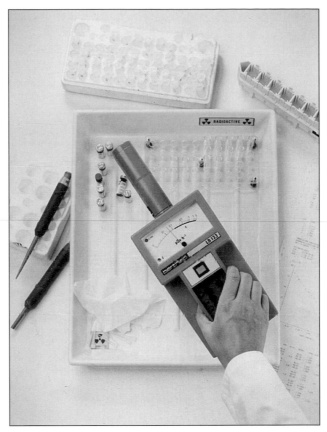

Fig. 7.19. Dose rate monitor (Berthold Instruments (UK) Ltd).

Method

1 Put on gloves and a laboratory coat and appropriate personal dosimeter.

2 Switch on monitor, allow to warm up and take background reading and other preliminary checks for battery conditions and checks with a known reference source.

3 Carefully and slowly sweep the probe as close as possible to the work surface to identify areas that give higher readings than background. Note readings at those areas when the needle or display has stabilised.

4 Record readings on sketch plan indicating the levels of contamination in the corresponding area.

5 Also monitor areas where contamination is most likely such as drawer or fridge handles, telephone.

6 Compare results with specified working derived limits or previous records.

Possible problems

1 The contaminating isotope must be known in order to select the most sensitive instrument.
2 Very low levels of contamination may be missed.

Swab or smear surveys

Smear surveys are an indirect method of measuring surface contamination levels. They are used either to detect soft β emitters and very low levels of contamination, or to monitor for contamination in an area of high radiation background.

To carry out a smear survey for tritium

Aim

The aim is to detect levels of contamination of soft β emitters such as tritium. Usually a contamination monitor cannot detect soft β emitters so they can only be monitored by frictional transfer.

Equipment required

A sketch plan of work areas, 25 mm Whatman GF disks, forceps, alcohol or other suitable liquid in a squeeze bottle, scintillation vials and liquid. 100 cm^2 templates (0.1 m^2).

Method

1 Put on gloves and laboratory coat and appropriate personal dosimeter.
2 Moisten the filter paper with alcohol and hold with forceps.
3 Put the template on a flat surface and uniformly wipe the work area with the moistened filter paper exposed within the template. Continue to sample as many areas as required using a fresh filter paper each time.
4 Fold the filter using the tips of forceps and place in labelled scintillation vial; cover with required amount of scintillation fluid.
5 Also swab possible contamination areas such as drawer handles and fridge handles where the template cannot be used.
6 Analyse in scintillation counter.
7 Calculate the contamination level (Bq m^{-2}) from

$$\text{Bq m}^{-2} = C_c \times \frac{100}{E_c} \times \frac{1}{A} \times \frac{100}{E_f}$$

where C_c = count rate in counts (corrected for background)

$\quad\quad E_c$ = overall percentage efficiency of the counting system

$\quad\quad A$ = area smeared or wiped in cm^2, and

$\quad\quad E_f$ = percentage of the contamination picked up by the filter paper. (This is difficult to determine as it is dependent on the physical and chemical nature of contamination, the nature of the base and so on. Usually a figure of 10 per cent is assumed unless known otherwise).

A quicker method employed in routine laboratories is to swab a large surface area using a damp paper towel and then to monitor the contamination picked up on the swab by an appropriate method. If the paper towel shows contamination then further monitoring should be carried out. This method also helps to keep work areas clean.

Air monitoring

As with airborne dust, certain types of radiation can be sampled on a filter paper using a high volume air sampler of the type shown in Fig. 7.20. A known volume of air is drawn through a filter, which is removed at the end of the sampling period and scanned for its radioactivity using a counter.

Particulate or gaseous airborne activity is measured by the filtration method described in Chapter 1. An appropriate filter paper is Whatman glass fibre for particles. Filters can also be impregnated with an agent such as charcoal for selective monitoring (including gases). These filters are usually placed in an open-face holder. The

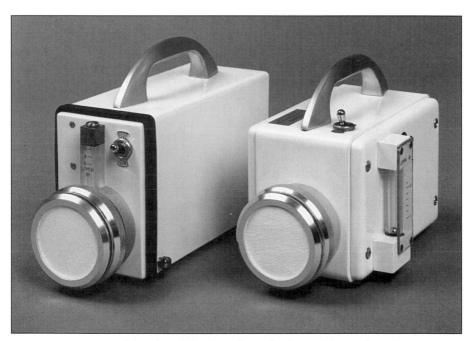

Fig. 7.20. High volume air samplers (Negretti Automation Ltd).

filter paper is then counted in a low background area directly with an appropriate detector or in the same way as for smear survey papers. The level of airborne contamination is calculated from:

$$\text{Bq m}^{-3} = C_c \times \frac{100}{E_c} \times \frac{1}{V},$$

where C_c = corrected count rate in counts per second

E_c = overall percentage efficiency of the counting system, and

V = volume of sampled air in cubic metres.

Radioactive gases that cannot be absorbed on impregnated filters can be measured by drawing a known volume of air into an appropriate sample bag or chamber which is filtered to remove particulate activity and then sealed. The sample is counted by an appropriate method in a low background and the gaseous activity calculated using the formula given above.

Biological monitoring

This is carried out in special circumstances and includes blood, urine or hair sampling. Thyroid monitoring can be carried out for iodine workers. Advice must be obtained as interpretation of results requires expert knowledge of the metabolic activities of the chemicals in question and its deposition preferences in the body.

Personal monitoring for external dose

There are three commonly used devices for monitoring external dose received by the individual. They are:

1 Film badge dosimeters.
2 Thermoluminescent dosimeters (TLD).
3 A direct reading device such as a pocket ionisation dosimeter or quartz-fibre electroscope (see Figs 7.16–7.18).

Personal monitoring with a film badge or TLD is usually undertaken by an Approved Dosimetry Service (approved by the HSE). Each dosimeter is numbered and is for use by one person only. The length of each monitoring period depends on the doses likely to be received during the period. Normally a dosimeter is worn for 4 weeks, but periods vary from 1 day, 1 week, 2 weeks to 3 months depending on type of dosimeter used and circumstances of work and nuclides handled.

The dosimeter is normally worn on the trunk at chest or waist height. The main concern is with the whole-body dose from external radiation. Film badges and body TLDs are worn with the label (open window) facing away from the body. For finger or wrist doses, the extremity TLD must be turned toward the area of highest potential dose. If there is any reason to suspect that doses to other parts of the body such as fingers or eyes may be received, extremity TLDs may be required as well as whole-body dosimeters. If protective clothing such as an apron is worn, the dosimeter is usually worn on the trunk under the apron. A dosimeter is also worn on the unprotected parts of the body if there is likely to be an exposure. Some examples of the various types of personal dosimeters are shown in Fig. 7.21.

Film badge dosimeter

A film sensitive to radiation is housed in a specially designed plastic casing containing windows of various materials, which shield certain kinds of radiation but which allow others to pass through. The device is worn during periods of exposure; one badge usually lasts a week or longer. The film is sent away to be developed and analysed for the accumulated dose of the various types of radiation. A permanent record of the employee's personal exposure is made.

Where exposure is from external sources such as X-rays, γ-rays (e.g. from caesium-137, iodine-125 and iodine-131) and high energy β-emitters (e.g. phosphorus-32) personal monitoring is widely carried out by means of a film badge. The dosimeter must be worn all the time when working with ionising radiation as it is monitoring an integrated dose to the whole body. This is true only if the wearer is in a uniform radiation field, which is rarely found in practice. In particular, work close to small sources or with narrow beams of radiation (e.g. X-ray crystallography, electron

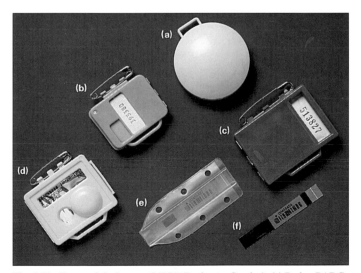

Fig. 7.21. Personal dosimeters (NRPB Dosimetry Service). (a) Radon PADC. (b) Film badge holder. (c) Thermoluminescent body badge holder. (d) Neutron film badge holder. (e) Thermoluminescent dosimeter finger strap in finger stall. (f) Thermoluminescent finger strap.

microscopes, cracks in shielding) involves exposure to many non-uniform fields. In such cases there is no simple method of obtaining a more accurate estimate of the whole body dose.

Advantages
1   Inexpensive and easily available.
2   Capable of integrating doses over a wide range.
3   Able to measure different radiation types and energies.
4   The developed film can be stored to provide a permanent record which can be read again if required.

Disadvantages
1   It has an energy dependent response especially for low energy radiation.
2   Response varies with angle relative to incident radiation.
3   There is a latent image fading of the film, which limits the monitoring period (4 weeks is best).
4   When the dosimeter is not being worn, care should be taken to prevent it from being exposed inadvertently to ionising radiation.
5   It is sensitive to heat and humidity so, if subjected to these conditions, heat and humidity could affect the assessment of doses.

Thermoluminescent dosimeter
Some materials such as lithium fluoride can change to what is known as an 'excited' state when bombarded with ionising radiation. This state is reversed only on the application of heat when the crystals return to normal but with a measurable emission of light. Thus a small badge containing these crystals can be used as a dosimeter as the degree of irradiation can be related to the amount of light produced on heating. An advantage with this type of dosimeter is that it is small and its analysis can be quickly and automatically performed.

The use of TLD is increasing for external dose monitoring, in many cases replacing the film badge for whole-body dose. They are often used in combination with the film badge – a film badge for whole-body dose monitoring and an extremity TLD strap for finger dose monitoring.

Advantages
1   A wide dose integration range.
2   A more energy-independent response than film badges.
3   No appreciable latent image fading or angular response variation.
4   Not as sensitive to the effects of heat and humidity as film badges.

Disadvantages

1   More expensive than film badges.

2   Dose information is destroyed at read-out, which eliminates the possibility of a re-check of the dose at a later date.

3   The thermoluminescent crystals or powder can give erroneous readings if damaged or if they become dirty through careless handling.

Film badges or TLDs will not detect low energy β emitters with no significant bremsstrahlung* emission (e.g. tritium, carbon-14, sulphur-35) as they will not penetrate the outer casing.

Direct reading monitors

In situations where an immediate indication of X or γ dose rate is desirable, then a direct reading monitor is commonly employed. They are normally self-indicating on a calibrated scale or a digital read-out so that the dose can be assessed at any phase of an operation involving potentially high exposures. For example, a self-indicating pocket dosimeter, about the size of a fountain pen (see Figs 7.16 and 7.17), is useful for measuring doses in situations where the dose rate is high since they allow a continuous watch to be kept on the rate of accumulation of dose. It is a miniature quartz-fibre ionisation dosimeter, charged with a small battery unit and the dose received since it was switched on can be read at any time. Another useful type of instrument is the personal alarm monitor, which gives an audible warning when a pre-set threshold radiation level is reached. It is particularly useful in many non-uniform fields.

The direct reading instruments that give instantaneous levels of dose received are usually used in conjunction with the film badge or TLD, which provide the permanent record of radiation dose received by the individual.

Disadvantages

1   Must be calibrated with known dose levels.

2   Expensive.

3   Insensitive to low energy radiation.

4   Can lose sensitivity due to leakage.

5   Fragile, so are easily damaged.

---

*   When charged particles are slowed down very rapidly after shielding with high density material, they emit energy in the form of X-rays. This is known as bremsstrahlung (braking radiation) and is of particular importance in the case of β-radiation.

Calibration of a dose rate instrument and conversion of a contamination monitor

Aim
When assessing the external radiation hazard, instruments that do not perform to specification can give misleading results, which can be dangerous. This practical shows how a dose rate monitor can be checked (steps 1 to 9) and how to use a contamination monitor to obtain an estimate of dose when a dose rate monitor is not available (steps 10 to 12).

Equipment required
A radiation source (e.g. 4 MBq radium-226), long tongs, metre rule, dose rate monitor, contamination monitor, shielding, long bench covered in absorbent sheeting with plastic backing (e.g. Benchkote).

Method
1   Put on appropriate protective clothing and personal dosimeter.
2   Cover bench with Benchkote, absorbent side up.
3   Place the metre rule on the Benchkote and mark 10-cm intervals.
4   Using long tongs, place the source so that it stands at the zero end of the metre rule.
5   With the probe of the dose rate monitor pointing towards the source, place it at 10-cm intervals along the metre rule and note the dose rate at each position.
6   Record the dose rate for each position.
7   Return the source to its shield.
8   Calculate the theoretical dose rate for each distance measured from:

$$\text{Dose rate } (\mu\text{Sv h}^{-1}) = \frac{\text{activity of source (GBq)} \times \text{constant *}}{\text{square of distance from source (m}^2)}$$

9   Plot the observed results against the calculated ones to produce a calibration curve for the instrument.
10   Repeat the exercise with a contamination monitor by placing its probe at the same distances from the exposed source and note the count rate at each position.
11   Replace the source in its container.
12   Plot the observed or the noted dose rates against counts per second to obtain a conversion curve for the instrument.

---

* Specific γ-ray constant if applicable.

Possible problems

1   This practical is best carried out in a Controlled Area.
2   Ensure that there is no exposure to other people entering the area under a System of Work during the time that the source is exposed.

To monitor hands and laboratory coats for contamination

Aim

When working with unsealed sources it is likely that protective clothing such as a laboratory coat can become contaminated. Contamination can also be transferred onto the hands by removing gloves incorrectly or contamination may spread from work areas by handling contaminated articles.

Equipment required

Hand-held monitor with appropriate probe for isotopes to be detected (Figs 7.7–7.8, 7.10 and 7.13). Laboratory coat (spot contaminated with a trace of a β-emitting isotope such as phosphorus-32).

Method

1   Go to an area such as the entrance lobby to the work area when there is a low level of background radiation.
2   Note background radiation after checking and allowing the monitor to stabilise.
3   While wearing the laboratory coat scan it slowly and evenly, holding the sensitive area of the probe as close to the surface of the coat as possible. Pay special attention to cuffs, the front of the coat and the pocket areas.
4   Scan the front and back surfaces of the hands in a similar manner.
5   Record the value and position of any readings above background.

Possible problems

1   Monitoring is painstakingly slow and laborious if done carefully.
2   Care must be taken to ensure that the probe is not contaminated.
3   If readings are high on laboratory coat, make arrangements for safe disposal.

To estimate the thickness of material required to give adequate shielding for a stored radionuclide

Aim
To ensure the adequate shielding of radionuclides that emit radiation so that they can be safely carried or stored.

Equipment required
Dose rate monitor, a radioactive source emitting hard β or γ rays, perspex sheets or blocks, lead bricks, and a tape measure.

Method
1   Put on appropriate protective clothing and personal dosimeter.
2   Measure dose rate on surface of container of the source.
3   Calculate thickness of lead shielding required to reduce dose rate at surface to 1 μSv h^{-1}.
4   Place calculated thickness of shielding around source and monitor again to confirm if thickness is adequate.

Example

Isotope to be shielded is cobalt-60. Dose rate at surface	= 32 μSv h^{-1}.
Required dose rate at outer surface of shielding	= 1 μSv h^{-1}.
The lead half-value layer (HVL) for cobalt-60	= 12.5 mm.

It is required to reduce dose rate from 32 μSv h^{-1} to 1 μSv h^{-1}; i.e. by a factor of 32. To do this will require 5 half-value layers of lead ($2 \times 2 \times 2 \times 2 \times 2 = 32$).

Therefore 5 $\times$ 12.5 mm of lead are required	= 62.5 mm.

Possible problems
1   Work as quickly as possible when measuring the unshielded source to reduce dose received by operator.
2   When β radiation from a radioactive source impinges on shielding materials, bremsstrahlung is produced, so be aware of this secondary radiation, which may also require shielding with a different material such as perspex.

Non-ionising radiation
Non-ionising radiations make up most of the low energy or longer wavelength of the electromagnetic spectrum as shown in Fig. 7.1. They include radiowaves, ultraviolet radiation, visible and infrared, ultrasound, lasers and microwaves.

The wavelength and radiation intensity of ultraviolet and infrared light emissions are relevant in that their biological effects are mainly on the skin and eyes. Intensity can be difficult to measure because the measuring instrument must be sensitive to the wavelength of the emitted radiation. Maximum Permissible Exposure limits vary widely in the British Standards, depending on exposure duration and wavelength. Visible lasers with short pulse duration represent the worst case with an exposure limit of 5 J m^{-2} for lasers in the wavelength 400–1050 nm.

Ultrasound is used in cleaning procedures and, if emitted at a sufficiently high intensity and at the right frequency, it can cause damage although no authoritative standards have been set for safe exposure levels for eyes or ears.

Lasers cause damage because the energy is concentrated on a very small area and can burn the skin and parts of the eyes. Where the eye transmits the frequency, the dangers are especially high as the energy can be focused to very high-power densities and damage the especially sensitive retina. There may be no need to measure the intensity of emission as it is often known or can be calculated from the manufacturer's stated power of the device, though checks should be made if possible. Special attention must be paid to pulsed lasers as their average power can be low but the peak power can be extremely high.

Microwaves are used for heating and cooking in commercial, industrial and domestic premises. They are also emitted from radio and radar transmitters. Their measurement can be difficult because microwaves occur over a wide range of wavelengths and the instrument used must be sensitive to the wavelength emitted. Microwave ovens for cooking are common and leakage of energy will occur if the doors are improperly sealed or become damaged as a result of wear and tear. High absorption of microwave energy causes rapid local heating particularly if the material contains a high proportion of water, since the resonant frequency of water molecules is within the microwave range. Thus a substance in the path of a fugitive beam could be affected. Since human tissue is made up of a large proportion of water it is particularly sensitive. Most microwave ovens operate at a frequency of 2450 Hz and instruments are available to measure leakage around the seals of ovens at this frequency. The standard that applies in the USA, but which is often used in the UK, (measured in milliwatts per square centimetre) is 10 mW cm^{-2}. An emission exceeding 1 mW cm^{-2} measured around the seal of a microwave oven suggests it requires attention.

The energy (E) of an electromagnetic wave is inversely proportional to wave frequency, so the lower the frequency, the less dangerous will be the radiation. This can be expressed as:

E = constant (k) × frequency.

Overheating of body tissues is the main hazard associated with non-ionising radiation. The safety levels are based on the maximum amount of energy per second that can safely be dissipated by unit area of the body surface. This is called *power surface density* and is measured in Joules per second per square metre (J s^{-1} m^{-1}) or watts per square metre (W m^{-2}). Often the subunit milliwatts per square centimetre (mW cm^{-2}) is used.

When determining safety standards some of the general principles considered are:

1   (a)   No effects demonstrated;
     (b)   effects discernible but there is no change in functional efficiency;
     (c)   some stress is discernible but only within the limits of normal physiological compensation.

2   Certain parts of the body such as the cornea of the eye will require lower safety levels as it has a poor blood supply and therefore is unable to dissipate heat.

3   Some sources of non-ionising radiations are pulsed, so though the average power surface density may be low the peak or instantaneous value may be high enough to cause permanent damage, e.g. by burning a blind spot on the retina of the eye.

4   High absorption of microwave energy causes rapid local heating because human tissue is made up of large proportion of water and the resonant frequency of water molecules is within the microwave region.

Table 7.10 lists some common sources of non-ionising radiation.

Table 7.10. Common sources of non-ionising radiation

Ultraviolet	Laser emission	Microwaves
Sunshine	Medical and scientific	Ovens
Sun-ray lamps	equipment	Radar equipment
Ultraviolet	Communications systems	Communication systems
microscopes	Lasers for entertainment	Scientific equipment
Mercury lamps	Surveying	
Carbon arcs		
Stroboscopes		
Welding equipment		

Microwaves

Protection standards

The safety levels are based on the heating effect of the microwaves. This is dependent upon the power of the source, the frequency of the source, the thermal and electrical properties of the tissue, and the cooling processes available to the tissue.

Organs such as the eye, the gall bladder and parts of the gastrointestinal system are particularly at risk since relatively little blood circulates in these tissues to provide the required cooling effect. The maximum power surface density permitted for continuous exposure is 100 watts per square metre (100 W m^{-2}).

In the cases of pulsed sources or intermittent exposure, higher levels are accepted as they are absorbed for a shorter period of time. It is the total energy that can safely be received in a given time, and the unit of energy used is watt hour (W h) or 3600 Joules.

Generally, for pulsed sources the safety level is taken to be 10 watt hours per square metre (10 W h m^{-2}) over a period of 0.1 hours or 6 minutes. This is equivalent to an average value of 100 W m^{-2}, which corresponds to the continuous exposure.

For example, a worker can tolerate powers of:

100 W m^{-2} continuously, or
200 W m^{-2} for 3 min once every 6 min, or
300 W m^{-2} for 2 min once every 6 min, or
600 W m^{-2} for 1 min once every 6 min, and so on.

This is subject to a maximum power of about 600 W m^{-2}, which compares with 1000 W m^{-2} absorbed in strong sunlight.

Care is required in the selection of monitoring and functional equipment as different countries adopt different safety standards as shown in Table 7.11.

Table 7.11. Standards adopted by some countries

Country	Exposure (W m^{-2})		
	Continuous	Intermittent	Maximum
UK	100	10 per 0.1 h	500
USA	100	10 per 0.1 h	250
Poland, Sweden, Czechoslovakia and Canada	2	$Time = \dfrac{32}{(power\ surface\ density)^2}$ *	100
Russia	0.1	—	10

* Power surface density levels are set in units of watts per square metre.

To measure the leakage of a microwave oven

Aim

To measure the leakage of energy around the seal of a microwave oven. This may arise if the door is improperly sealed or the seals have become damaged accidentally or as a result of wear and tear.

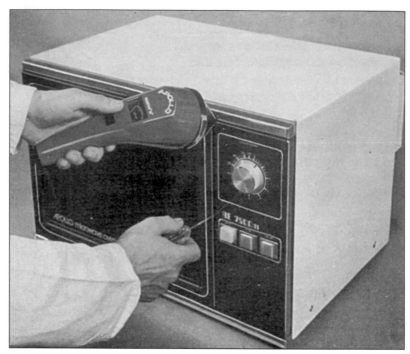

Fig. 7.22. Microwave monitor (Apollo Enterprises).

Equipment required
Microwave oven, microwave monitor, e.g. the 'Apollo N' (Fig. 7.22), a glass beaker containing 300 ml of a 0.1% aqueous solution.

Method
1   Place the beaker of water on the load-carrying surface of the oven after switching the oven on to full power.
2   Carry out the instrument checks as specified by the manufacturer.
3   Energise the monitor by depressing the black push-button as per instructions.
4   Zero the meter, keeping the switch depressed and pointing the monitor away from the source of radiation.
5   Move the monitor over the external surface of the oven, especially around the seal of the door to locate any points of microwave leakage. Read the field intensity directly in W m^{-2} from the scale on the monitor.
6   Release the push-button switch. This will automatically switch off the monitor.

Lasers

The retina of the eye is most at risk from laser radiation. This could arise by focusing the eye lens on the narrow beam.

Some properties of laser generators that are of interest are that they produce an intense, monochromatic beam of non-ionising electromagnetic radiation, the wavelengths of radiation emitted depend on the lasing medium, e.g. helium-neon gas, the output beams are of low angular divergence, and the output of continuous waves (cw) and pulsed waves is 10^{-12} $t < 0.25$ s.

Hazards from lasers arise from:

1   Skin exposure where thermal and photochemical damage may occur.

2   Optical imaging effects, which are critical in visible region. In the range 400 nm to 1400 nm the eye acts as a lens imaging system. Point images are produced on the retina about a million times as intense as the unfocused light incident on the cornea.

3   Hazards from electrical power supplies.

Lasers are categorised into the following classes:

Class I: Low power, emission well below maximum permissible exposure (MPE) level.

Class II: Low power, visible radiation (400–700 nm), for example ≤ 1 mW continuous wave laser.

Class IIIa: Output power ≤ 5 mW for continuous lasers of visible radiation.

Class IIIb: Output power ≤ 0.5 W continuous power and $\leq$ J m^{-2} for pulsed lasers, visible and invisible radiation emitted.

Class IV: High output capable of producing hazardous diffuse reflections.

Particular hazards from lasers to the body and safety precautions to take are shown in Tables 7.12 and 7.13.

For Class IIIa intrabeam viewing may be hazardous while Class IIIb lasers are usually viewed via a diffuse reflector to ensure that working distance is always greater than 50 mm, the viewing time less than 10 seconds and the diffuse image diameter greater than 5.5 mm.

Class IV lasers may cause skin injuries and can be fire hazards.

Table 7.12. Particular hazards from lasers to the body

Spectral region	Eye	Skin
Ultraviolet (200–280 nm)	Photokerevatitus	Erythema, pigmentation increased
Ultraviolet B (280–315 nm)	Photokeretitus	Erythema, pigmentation increased
Ultraviolet A (3.5–400 nm)	Photochemical cataract	Pigment darkening, photosensitive reactions
Visible (400–780 nm)	Photochemical injury, thermal retinal injury	Pigment darkening, photosensitive reactions
Infrared A (780–1400 nm)	Cataract burn, retinal burn	Skin burn
Infrared B (1.4–3 m)	Aqueous flare, cataract and cornea burn	Skin burn
Infrared C (3–1 mm)	Cornea burn	Skin burn

Table 7.13. Safety precautions when using lasers

Laser	1	2	3a	3b	4
Remote interlock	Not required		Connect to door		
Key control	Not required		Remove key when laser not in use		
Beam attenuator	Not required		Prevents inadvertent exposure		
Emission indicator	Not required		Indication required		
Warning signs	Not required	Provide signs plus precautions			
Beam termination	Not required	Terminate beam			
Specular reflection	No hazard	Care required	Prevent unwanted reflections		
Eye protection	No special precautions			Special precautions required	
Protective clothing	No special precautions			Sometimes required	Recommend
Training	Not necessary		Required for all users		

Dose units for lasers

The dose received from a continuous wave laser is measured in power surface density in watts per square centimetre (W cm^{-2}) and from pulsed lasers in energy surface density per pulse in Joules per square centimetre (J cm^{-2}) per pulse.

Maximum permissible exposure (MPE) levels are imposed at:

1 *Constant power (W m^{-2}) levels* are applied at long exposure and very short exposure times.

2 *Constant energy (J m^{-2}) levels* are applied at short exposure times for wavelengths greater than 400 nm. In the ultraviolet and visible it applies at longer exposure times of greater than 10 seconds.

The safety standards for MPE levels are detailed in the British Standard BS 4803:1972 and are complex to interpret. The conditions are given for laser exposure for wavelength range 200 nm–1 mm and for the exposure times of 0–3 × 10^4 seconds. They also include cases for intrabeam viewing, extended source viewing, skin exposure for continuous wave, pulsed and multi-pulsed conditions.

Ultraviolet radiation

Usually ultraviolet radiation is subdivided into three regions:

Ultraviolet A (UV A): wavelength 400–315 nm
Ultraviolet B (UV B): wavelength 315–280 nm
Ultraviolet C (UV C): wavelength 280–100 nm

Wavelengths below 200 nm are attenuated by the atmosphere so are not considered to be a hazard. Above approximately 200 nm the eyes and skin can be at risk to over-exposure.

Hazards

The eyes suffer from kerato-conjunctivitis, sometimes called 'arc eye' or 'welder's flash' or 'snow blindness'. The symptoms are pain as if having grit in the eye and an aversion to bright lights. The symptoms do not cause permanent damage and usually disappear after about 36 hours of rest.

The skin suffers from sunburn or erythema (which is reddening of the skin) mainly produced by ultraviolet B radiation.

Dose and exposure standards

The UK follows the guidelines laid down in the USA or the guidelines laid down by the International Non-Ionising Radiation Committee (INIRC) of the International Radiation Protection Association (IRPA), shown in Tables 7.14 and 7.15. Doses are in Joules per unit area for an 8-hour period.

As the values given in Table 7.14 apply only to sources emitting essentially monochromatic ultraviolet radiation, a calculation must be made to assess the effective irradiance of a broad-band source. The MPE for a broad-band source is calculated by summing the relative contributions from all its spectral components, each contribution being weighted by the relative spectral effectiveness.

$$E_{eff} = E_\lambda + S_\lambda + \Delta_\lambda$$

where E_{eff} = effective irradiance relative to monochromatic wavelength 270 nm (W m^{-2})

$\quad\quad E_\lambda$ = spectral irradiance at wavelength (W m^{-2} nm^{-1})

$\quad\quad S_\lambda$ = relative spectral effectiveness of radiation of wavelength, and

$\quad\quad \Delta_\lambda$ = band width employed in the measurements or calculation of E_λ (nm).

The MPE, expressed in seconds, may be calculated by dividing the MPE for 270 nm radiation (30 J m^{-2}) by the effective irradiance (W m^{-2}). Values of MPE are given in Table 7.15.

Table 7.14. Ultraviolet radiation exposure limits and spectral weighing function; IRPA/INIRC 1988 Revision

Wavelength* (nm)	Exposure limit (J m^{-2})	–Exposure limit (mJ cm^{-2})	Relative spectral effectiveness (S)
180	2.500	250	0.012
190	1.600	160	0.019
200	1.000	100	0.030
205	590	59	0.051
210	400	40	0.075
215	320	32	0.095
220	250	25	0.120
225	200	20	0.150
230	160	16	0.190
235	130	13	0.240
240	100	20	0.300
245	83	8.3	0.360
250	70	7.0	0.430
254†	60	6.0	0.500
255	58	5.8	0.520
260	46	4.6	0.650
265	37	3.7	0.810
270	30	3.0	1.000
275	31	3.1	0.960
280	34	3.4	0.880
285	39	3.9	0.770

Table 7.14. (cont.)

Wavelength* (nm)	Exposure limit (J m^{-2})	Exposure limit (mJ cm^{-2})	Relative spectral effectiveness (S)
290	47	4.7	0.640
295	56	5.6	0.540
297†	65	6.5	0.460
300	100	10	0.300
303†	250	25	0.190
305	500	50	0.060
308	1.200	120	0.026
310	2.000	200	0.015
313	5.000	500	0.006
315	1.0×10^4	1.0×10^3	0.003
316	1.3×10^4	1.3×10^3	0.0024
317	1.5×10^4	1.5×10^3	0.0020
318	1.9×10^4	1.9×10^3	0.0016
319	2.5×10^4	2.5×10^3	0.0012
320	2.9×10^4	2.9×10^3	0.0010
322	4.5×10^4	4.5×10^3	0.00067
323	5.6×10^4	5.6×10^3	0.00054
325	6.0×10^4	6.0×10^3	0.00050
328	6.8×10^4	6.8×10^3	0.00044
330	7.3×10^4	7.3×10^3	0.00041
333	8.1×10^4	8.1×10^3	0.00037
335	8.8×10^4	8.8×10^3	0.00034
340	1.1×10^5	1.1×10^4	0.00028
345	1.3×10^5	1.5×10^4	0.00024
350	1.5×10^5	1.5×10^4	0.00020
355	1.9×10^5	1.9×10^4	0.00016
360	2.3×10^5	2.3×10^4	0.00013
365	2.7×10^5	2.7×10^4	0.00011
370	3.2×10^5	3.2×10^4	0.000093
375	3.9×10^5	3.9×10^4	0.000077
380	4.7×10^5	4.7×10^4	0.000064
385	5.7×10^5	5.7×10^4	0.000053
390	6.8×10^5	6.8×10^4	0.000044
395	8.3×10^5	8.3×10^4	0.000036
400	1.0×10^6	1.0×10^5	0.000030

* Wavelengths chosen are representative; other values should be interpolated at intermediate wavelengths.
† Emission lines of a mercury discharge spectrum.

It is important that the contribution of all wavelengths emitted by the source is taken into account. This has the effect of reducing the permitted exposure to below that for 8 hours.

Table 7.15. Maximum permissible exposures in an 8-hour period

Effective irradiance relative to monochromatic wavelength 270 nm (W m^{-2})	Maximum permissible exposures
10^3	8 (h)
8×10^{-3}	1 (h)
5×10^{-2}	10 (min)
5×10^{-1}	1 (min)
3	10 (s)
30	1 (s)
3×10^2	0.1 (s)

The MPE expressed in seconds may be calculated by dividing the MPE for 270 nm radiation (30 J m^{-2}) by E_{eff} (W m^{-2}).

Protective measures

Protective measures are more important than monitoring. Some of these will include:

Appropriate eye protection.
Interlocks for areas of high radiation.
Systems of work.
Labelling of sources.
Warning lights.
Safety enclosures for sources.

There are also other physical hazards associated with non-ionising radiation equipment. For example, many ultraviolet lamps are charged at a high pressure, so care should be taken in handling them to prevent an explosion. Lasers usually require high voltage power supplies for their operation.

References and further reading

Ionising radiation

Code of Practice for Site Radiography (1975) Kluwer-Harrop, London.
Department of the Environment (1970) *Code of Practice for the Carriage of Radioactive Materials by Road.* HMSO, London.
Department of Health and Social Security (1972) *Code of Practice for the Protection of Persons Against Ionising Radiation Arising from Medical and Dental Use.* HMSO, London.
Doran, D. (1980) Ionising radiation: physics, measurement, control. In: *Occupational Hygiene* (eds H.A. Waldron & J.M. Harrington), pp. 280–300. Blackwell Scientific Publications, Oxford.
Ennis, J.R. (1987) New dosimetry at Hiroshima and Nagasaki – implications for risk estimates. *NRPB Radiological Bulletin* **85**, 24–27.
European Community (1984) *Official Journal of the European Communities.* L246, 17 September 1980, and L265, 5 October 1984.

Faires, R.A. & Boswell, G.G.J. (1987) *Radioisotope Laboratory Techniques,* 4th edn. Butterworths, London.

Guidance Notes for the Protection of Persons Exposed to Ionising Radiation in Research and Teaching (1977) HMSO, London.

Health and Safety Executive (1985) *Approved Code of Practice for the Protection of Persons Against Ionising Radiation Arising from any Work Activity.* HMSO, London.

Health and Safety Executive (1989) *Radiation Safety for Operators of Gamma Irradiation Plants.* UK Panel on Gamma and Electron Irradiation. HMSO, London.

Health and Safety at Work etc. Act, 1984. HMSO, London.

International Commission on Radiation Units and Measurements (1971) *Radiation Protection Instrumentation and its Application.* Report 20. ICRP, Washington DC.

International Commission on Radiological Protection (1977) *Recommendations of the International Commission on Radiological Protection.* Publication 26, Annuals of the ICRP, Vol. 1, No. 3. Pergamon Press, Oxford.

Ionising Radiation (Unsealed Radioactive Substances) Regulations (1985) HMSO, London.

Ionising Radiations (Sealed Sources) Regulations (1969) HMSO, London.

Martin, A. & Harbison, S.A. (1988) *An Introduction to Radiation Protection,* 2nd edn. Chapman & Hall, London.

National Radiological Protection Board (1988) *Living with Radiation.* NRPB, Didcot.

Nuclear Installations Act, 1965. HMSO, London.

Nuclear Installations Act, 1969. HMSO, London.

Radioactive Substances Act, 1960. HMSO, London.

Radioactive Substances Act, 1960 (1963) An explanatory memorandum for persons keeping or using radioactive materials. HMSO, London.

Radioactive Substances (Carriage by Road) (Great Britain) Regulations (1970) HMSO, London.

Radioactive Substances (Road Transport Workers) (Great Britain) Regulations (1970) HMSO, London.

The Factories Act, 1961. HMSO, London.

The Ionising and Radiations Regulations (1985) HMSO, London.

The Radiochemical Manual, 2nd edn. Amersham International, Amersham (out of print).

Non-ionising radiation

General

Kanagasabay, S. (1980) Non-ionising radiation. In: *Occupational Hygiene* (eds H.A. Waldron & J.M. Harrington), pp. 257–279. Blackwell Scientific Publications, Oxford.

Microwaves

American National Standards Institution. *Safety Level of Electromagnetic Radiation with Respect of Personnel.* C 95.1. ANSI. (Updated regularly.)

Medical Research Council (1971) *Exposure to Microwave and Radiofrequency Radiation.* MRC/170/1314, London.

Safety Precautions Relating to Intense Radiofrequency Radiation (1974) HMSO, London.

Lasers

American National Standards Institution (1976) *American National Standard for the Safe Use of Lasers.* ANSI 2136.1.

BSI Standards (1972) *Protection of Persons against Hazards from Laser Radiation.* BS 4803. BSI Standards, Milton Keynes.

BSI Standards (1982) *Radiation Safety of Laser Products and Systems.* BS 4803. BSI Standards, Milton Keynes. (Part 1: General; Part 2: Specification for Manufacturing Requirements for Laser Products; Part 3: Guidance for Users.)

Department of Education and Science (1970) *The Use of Lasers in Schools and Other Educational Establishments.* Administrative Memorandum 7170. HMSO, London.

Ultraviolet radiation

American Conference of Governmental Industrial Hygienists (1998) *Threshold Limit Values for Chemical Substances and Physical Agents and Biological Exposure Indices (BEIs).* ACGIH, Cincinnati.

Department of Health, Education and Welfare (NIOSH) (1972) *Criteria for a Recommended Standard–Occupational Exposure to Ultra-violet Radiation.* Publication No. 73–1100. DHEW (NIOSH), Cincinnati.

McKinlay, A.F. & Diffey, B.L. (1987) A reference action spectrum for ultra-violet induced erythema in human skin. In: *Human Exposure to Ultra-violet Radiation: Risks and Regulations*, Proceedings of a seminar held in Amsterdam 23–25 March 1987 (eds W.F. Passchier & B.F.M. Bosnjakovic). Elsevier Science Publishers, Amsterdam.

National Radiological Protection Board (1977) *Protection Against Ultra-violet Radiation in the Workplace.* HMSO, London.

Parrish, J.A., Jaenicke, K.F. & Anderson, R.R. (1982) Erythema and melanogenesis action spectra of normal human skin. *Photochemistry and Photobiology* **36**(2), 187–191.

Urbach, F. & Gange, R.W. (1986) *The Biological Effects of UVA Radiation.* Praeger Publications, New York.

8 Microbiological hazards

Introduction

Micro-organisms have always been used at the domestic and industrial level in activities such as brewing, baking, pickling, cheese and yoghurt manufacture, wine making and in the selective breeding of plants and animals. A major part of monitoring for microbial or microbiological hazards, originally called bacterial hazards, in certain industries such as food products, and chemical and pharmaceutical industries, is undertaken for quality control or quality assurance purposes. Examples of this include the purity of raw materials, contamination of products, and to ensure sterility of the workplace and equipment. Microbial monitoring is also undertaken in the agricultural industry to prevent or control certain diseases in animals or poultry. However, with the increase in work with pathogens and the advent of new biotechnological innovations for large-scale production of novel substances and legislation such as the Control of Substances Hazardous to Health, 1988 and the Genetic Manipulation Regulations, 1990, the need for microbiological monitoring in the workplace is becoming more important to health and safety professionals.

The work areas where the risk of infection is high are biological laboratories in industry and research institutions, diagnostic laboratories in hospitals and production areas of biological materials. The risk could arise from handling animal or human tissue such as post-mortem materials, blood, cultures, solutions, reagents, etc., which may contain harmful strains of these microbes. It is therefore imperative that anyone working in these areas knows the potential microbiological hazards, where to seek expert advice and the statutory controls required in the use of certain microbes. All procedures must be safe, work areas clearly designated and protected against contamination, and all equipment safeguarded.

Though most micro-organisms are harmless free-living or soprophytic bacteria or fungi that pose no threat to human health, they can create expensive contamination problems that can at times be difficult to control. However, there are a few microbes that are highly infectious for humans. In many cases micro-organisms have simple nutritional requirements and can develop resistance to imposed stresses.

As different micro-organisms vary in their ability to cause ill-health they are classified into hazard groups. The classification is based on the risk to employees in the route they can use to produce human infection and also to the community if the organisms escape the work area. The hazard group in which an organism is placed determines the extent of precautions that are necessary for its culture and use.

The Advisory Committee on Dangerous Pathogens (ACDP) classifies micro-organisms according to the following criteria:

1   Is the organism pathogenic or disease-producing to man?
2   Is it a hazard to employees?
3   Is it transmissible in the community?
4   Is effective prophylaxis and treatment available?

There are four hazard groups. The hazard group in which an organism is placed determines the precautions required for its use or culture. The more hazardous the micro-organisms, the more stringent the precautions necessary for handling them safely. The precautions required are the four containment or biosafety levels. These are also given numbers that correspond to the hazard group numbers. Most micro-organisms used generally are in Hazard Group 1 and are considered to be harmless. Usually the precautions taken to avoid contamination and purity of the product, known as good manufacturing practice (GMP) or good large scale practice (GLSP), would offer sufficient protection to the employees. However, some micro-organisms are in Group 2 and a few in Group 3 where the precautions taken are more stringent.

• *Group 1*: An organism that is most unlikely to cause human disease.

• *Group 2*: An organism that may cause human disease and which might be a hazard to employees but is unlikely to spread in the community. Exposure at work rarely produces specific infection and effective treatment or prophylaxis is readily available.

• *Group 3*: An organism that may cause severe human disease and present a severe hazard to employees. It may present a high risk of spread in the community but there is usually effective prophylaxis or treatment available.

• *Group 4*: An organism that causes severe human disease and is a serious hazard to employees. It may present a high risk of spread in the community and there is usually no effective prophylaxis treatment.

The groups, other than Group 1, are referred to as *pathogens* and the organisms in Group 4 are known as *listed pathogens*.

Micro-organisms, besides possibly being pathogenic, can be hazardous to the health of the people who work with them. For example, some microbial toxins could have their hazardous potential increased when grown under artificial conditions. The infectivity of strains is often related to dose received and mode of entry into the body, as well as to the health status and resistance to disease of the employees.

In addition to these potential hazards from natural micro-organisms, there are also perceived hazards from genetically modified micro-organisms. Genetic materials from one organism can be inserted into another to obtain higher or purer yields of vaccines, therapeutic substances and useful chemicals. The concern is from errors in production or release of micro-organisms for which there is no effective treatment.

Principles of containment

To prevent micro-organisms from entering into or infecting a worker or the work area, various levels of barriers need to be set up:

1   Primary barriers are used to confine the organisms so that they cannot escape from the containers in which they are produced or handled. This is done by the use of appropriate equipment including microbiological safety cabinets and by the use of effective disinfection and sterilisation procedures and by good laboratory and industrial practice.

2   Secondary barriers are the barriers that are placed between the worker and the organisms. These include protective clothing, medical surveillance and immunisation and a high level of personal hygiene.

3   Tertiary barriers are placed around the work areas, which includes security and limited access, supervision of invitees and visitors. They also include procedures such as autoclaving of infected waste before it leaves the work areas and waste management.

Work with microbes is normally confined to specifically designated work areas. Ideally these work areas should be provided with a ventilation system for which the air supplied to the corridors always flows into the work areas and in which there is a slight excess of exhaust over supply, which creates 'negative' pressure. Although circumstances vary according to needs, the air is often filtered both at the inlet and exhaust ends of the system and where necessary, forced by a fan through high-efficiency particulate air (HEPA) filters.

Micro-organisms

Micro-organisms are individual plants or animals that are too small to be visible to the naked eye. Like dust, micro-organisms are ubiquitous, though the majority of them are harmless and some are even beneficial to man.

Specific definitions and detailed descriptions are available in the literature and it is recommended that the reader consults a good textbook before any monitoring is carried out in order to understand the basic principles of the behaviour of micro-organisms and procedures for their detection.

Viruses

These are submicroscopic (below the magnification power of the light microscope) particles, ranging in size from 20 to 450 nm in diameter and are not truly living organisms. Viruses consist of the genetic materials deoxyribonucleic acid (DNA) or ribonucleic acid (RNA) surrounded by a protein coat and possibly other components, and they can reproduce and replicate only in other living cells. Although viruses may be present in the work environment, they will die or remain dormant until a suitable living cell is available for their reproduction to commence and progress. The genetic material is enclosed in virions, varying in size from 100 to 1000 nm, which are capsules or coats of protein and/or lipids. Viruses can be the cause of diseases in certain specialised industries only, for example in farming, veterinary work and the pharmaceutical industry.

Some RNA viruses contain oncogenes. These genes are capable of initiating tumours in animals.

Bacteria

Bacteria are free-living single cells with an average size of 0.5 μm, and are capable of reproducing themselves when they grow on solid or semi-solid surfaces that provide their nutrients. They do not need other cells for their survival. They are found in different forms or colonies which are visible as:

cocci (spheres), which form clumps, pairs or chains,
bacilli (rods),
spirochaetes (spirals or filamentous),
actinomycetes (long rods that may show branching).

They have two types of cell wall. This affects their capacity to retain stains (Gram positive and negative) offering a method for their identification (Table 8.1). Many bacteria form spores or resistant dormant forms. This has a bearing on their ability to survive under various environmental conditions and contribute to their classification.

Table 8.1. Examples of types of bacteria

	Cocci	Rods
Gram positive	*Staphylococcus aureus*	*Lactobacillus*
	Streptococcus faecalis	*Corynebacterium*
	Micrococcus lutes	
Gram negative	*Neisseria vaginalis*	*Salmonella*
		Escherichia coli
		Pseudomonas aeruginosa

Bacteria are prokaryotes, that is, they do not have a defined nucleus and the genetic material is not seen clearly, as distinct from eukaryotes, that is, higher forms of life which have a definite nucleus inside a nuclear membrane.

Bacteria are ubiquitous in many environments and reproduce very freely. Bacteria, like yeast and moulds, need water to reproduce so they do not reproduce in air although it is used extensively as a transport medium. Some have flagella, which enable them to move through liquids.

Bacteria can reproduce asexually by dividing into two (binary fission). Each environment or habitat supports specialised types of bacteria. Each is adapted to make the best of that environment, which helps in their identification. For example, Gram-negative rods are sensitive to drying so are usually found only in moist or wet habitats. Gram-positive cocci, on the other hand, are associated with animal skins and mucous membranes. The majority of bacteria are harmless and many are beneficial though some species can be pathogenic under specific circumstances.

Because of the ubiquitous nature of bacteria, a source of bacterial contamination is difficult to identify. In industries whose products are ingested by humans, everything in the work area is usually monitored so that the level of micro-organisms on products at all stages of preparation is known and so the risk to employees can be estimated. Tables 8.2–8.4 give examples of active, passive and surface sampling methods. To reduce the level of routine monitoring, micro-organisms are kept to a minimum by various procedures. These include treatment of the raw materials to reduce the number of micro-organisms to an acceptable level, regular washing and sterilisation of equipment, purification and distribution of water in-house to the standards required, filtering of air, enclosure of work processes, and wearing of sterile clothing during work.

Bacteria may vary in their resistance to adverse physical conditions such as high or low temperatures and pressures and ultrasound. Therefore, the methods used to destroy them must be selected with care. For example, for those species that cannot survive at 100 °C for more than a few minutes, autoclaving may be the appropriate method for sterilising the articles used. The type of disinfectant, concentration and contact time can be critical too.

The measures taken to destroy or disable bacteria will usually kill or disable yeasts, moulds and viruses. Yeasts and moulds are generally not pathogenic to man but are important from a spoilage point of view.

Mycoplasma are bacteria that have no defined cell walls. They are variable in shape and can pass through bacteria-excluding filters because they can change their shape to fit the filter pore size.

Table 8.2. Examples of active sampling

Method of sampling	Advantages	Disadvantages	Manufacturer
Slit to agar	Very efficient Samples large volumes Plates directly incubated	Bulky Adjustment critical May dry out	Casella, Raynier
Sieve and cascade samples	Efficient Non-intrusive Plate directly incubated	Single stage Large numbers of particles expelled	Anderson, SAS, Casella
Centrifugal	Portable Strips directly incubated	Sample volume not known Strips supplied by one manufacturer only	Abinghurst Biotest
Liquid	Very efficient Total numbers of organisms in sample can be determined	Clumsy Needs plating out Fragile	Millipore, Casella
Filtration membrane	Efficient Samples large volumes	Dries and kills organisms Needs plating out	Casella, Millipore, Gelman, Sartorius
Gelatine	Efficient Samples large volumes May give total number of organisms in unit volume	Needs plating out	In-house or purchased from Sartorius

Table 8.3. Examples of passive sampling

Methods of sampling	Advantages	Disadvantages	Manufacturer
Settle plates	Cheap Easy to use	Sampling volumes not known May dry out	Sartorius
Broth runs	Predicts actual contamination rate Good validation exercise	Expensive in production time Difficult to evaluate	Sartorius

Note: all require aspectic techniques and practice.

Table 8.4. Examples of surface sampling

Methods of sampling	Advantages	Disadvantages	Manufacturer
Surface swab	Cheap Easy	Relies on frictional transfer, efficiency poor Qualitative	
Contact plates	Cheap Easy Semi-quantitative	Relies on adhesion 20–70% efficient Leaves nutrient film behind	Radoc, Sartorius
Finger dabs	Cheap Easy Semi-quantitative	Relies on transfer, efficiency poor	Radoc, Sartorius
Agar overlay	Very efficient Quantitative	Clumsy Needs supply of inert strips	Radoc, Sartorius

Note: all require aspectic techniques and practice.

Rickettsia, Chlamydia and *Coxiella* are small bacteria that reproduce by division and live and reproduce in animal cells.

Commensals are micro-organisms that live in or on a human body. They do not cause any inconvenience or disease and many are capable of an independent existence, for example the flora in the human gut.

Pyrogens are fever-producing compounds that increase body temperatures when ingested. An example is endotoxins, which are fragments from the cell walls of Gram-negative bacteria.

Yeasts
Yeasts are usually bigger than bacteria and have their nuclear materials in a cell nucleus, whereas bacterial nuclear material is free in the cytoplasm. Yeasts are usually reproduced by budding.

Moulds
Moulds are microscopic plants with projections called mycelia. These can be broken into pieces that will grow larger and reproduce. They also produce spores, which become airborne but are not as resistant as bacterial spores. Moulds vary in their resistance to adverse conditions such as low pH and higher concentration of disinfectant.

Yeasts and moulds are found more often in dust and therefore can be picked up in air samples since they are more resistant to drying than bacteria.

Bacteriophages

Bacteriophages are special viruses capable of infecting bacteria and this property is used in genetic engineering, manipulation or modification. In simple terms, genetic modification is the incorporation of nucleic acid from one source into another. The bacteriophage is also known as a carrier, which can be a virus or bacterial plasmid. This allows the incorporation of genetic material into an organism in which it does not exist naturally but where it can survive and reproduce. Under certain conditions such plasmids can be incorporated into new cells. Alternatively, DNA can be incorporated into bacteriophages, which can then transfer the DNA to a new cell.

Monitoring techniques

Many operations in work areas produce airborne micro-organisms. Some of these include the use of hypodermic syringes, wire loops, centrifuges, cultures, ampoules, maceration, homogenising, sonicating, shaking, spray drying and pipetting. Bacterial spores and moulds can travel as free entities in air currents. Some organisms are transferred by associating with something else like skin scales or droplets of liquids. Other mechanisms of transfer include touch, either person to article, article to article or contact with contaminated fluid such as water or too dilute disinfectant. Scrupulous sterility is essential to keep to a minimum unwanted micro-organisms that would otherwise proliferate in any appropriate growth medium.

Monitoring for microbiological hazards, like other forms of monitoring, entails various stages. The monitoring stages include taking a representative sample, examining or analysing it and interpreting the results before any conclusions can be drawn.

Taking samples can be carried out by the health and safety professional under the guidance of a microbiologist or quality control expert. The people who take the samples, however, must be trained in aseptic techniques. They must understand the routes by which the samples can become contaminated and therefore become invalid. The methods of monitoring will depend on the objectives for which monitoring is undertaken.

As mentioned before, in a comprehensive monitoring programme the raw materials, water, the final product and the environment are monitored involving many specialists.

Handling micro-organisms

Micro-organism cultures must always be handled carefully, as if they contained pathogens. Work with micro-organisms can be performed safely if the following safety rules are observed:

- Wash hands thoroughly before and after working.

- Do not eat or drink in the work area.

- Do not touch known micro-organisms with the hands.

- Never pipette suspensions containing micro-organisms with the mouth. Always use mechanical aids to pipette (e.g. Peleus ball).

- Prior to and after use, sterilise inoculating loops and wires by flaming until they glow red-hot.

- Sterilise all equipment that comes in contact with micro-organisms.

- Ensure that everything that leaves the work area is not infectious by disinfecting, autoclaving or incineration.

As mentioned before, it is sometimes necessary to monitor not only the kinds of micro-organisms present in materials to be handled, but also the number of micro-organisms. These include total counts and viable counts, for which plate counts and membrane filter counts are most frequently used along with the dip slide method for liquids.

When total counts are undertaken, both dead and living organisms are included in the count. It is difficult to distinguish between the debris and the microbes so this count is of limited value. In one method, a known amount of liquid or emulsified solid is spread onto a microscope slide, stained, and then examined with a microscope that has a glass graticule with a grid of squares of known size. The organisms are counted in a suitable number of squares and the total count for unit volume is then calculated. In another method, the counting chamber uses a slide with a recess of known depth on which a grid is engraved. The material to be examined, usually a liquid, is placed in the recess, covered with a cover slip and examined under a microscope. The organisms are counted in an appropriate number of squares and the number of organisms per unit volume is calculated since the depth of fluid and the area of squares are known.

Total viable counts originally known as bacterial counts are used for organisms that are alive and capable of growing on selected media. For the plate count the sample is homogenised in a sterile dilutent and several dilutions of the sample – e.g. 1:10, 1:100 or 1:1000 – are made. Known volumes of the sample are placed in

Petri dishes, then melted agar culture medium is poured in the dishes and mixed with the sample. After the agar has set solid the dishes are incubated for 24–48 hours. The numbers of colonies that grow are counted and represent the numbers of colony-forming viable units in that sample; the results are usually expressed as viable counts per ml or gram. For the membrane filter counts, a thin cellulose acetate film made to precise specifications is used as a filter to retain microbes. The microbes are retained on its surface, which is ruled in squares of known area.

The membrane is supported in a filter apparatus and a known volume of the sample, suitably diluted where appropriate, is sucked or pushed through under pressure. The membrane is then incubated after being placed on an absorbent pad soaked in liquid culture medium. The number of colonies that grow are counted and represent the number of viable colony-forming units per ml or gram of the sample. Plate counts can only be done in a laboratory but membranes can be used in the field and then incubated in the laboratory.

The membrane can also be treated with a fluorescent stain that is known to be taken up by the living organisms. The unabsorbed stain is washed away and the membrane examined under the microscope under special conditions incorporating ultraviolet light. The microbes become fluorescent, usually green or orange, and are then counted in the squares.

The dip slide is a flat plastic strip 5 cm long and 2 cm wide and 3 mm deep, which is separated into a number of squares containing agar culture medium. It is attached to the underside of a cap which screws on to a glass bottle. When required the slide is dipped into the fluid to be examined, returned to the bottle and sealed, incubated and the colonies counted. Various culture media slides are available so a range of organisms can be counted by this method.

Atmospheric sampling for micro-organisms can be either *active* or *passive*. Active sampling (Table 8.2) involves drawing a sample of air through a collection device and subsequently analysing the collected sample. An example of an active sample is given in Figs 8.1 and 8.2. Size selection can be achieved by means of a cascade impacter as shown in Fig. 8.2. Passive sampling (Table 8.3) involves allowing the micro-organisms from the workroom air to settle on a collecting device (Fig. 8.3). After collection the sample is incubated at an appropriate temperature. Total viable colonies are then counted using a colony counter as shown in Fig. 8.4.

The main methods of surface sampling are shown in Table 8.4. Sample locations are important. Examples of these could be the dirtiest point in a room or a product at highest risk. In industries that handle micro-organisms, it is important to sample the air in the

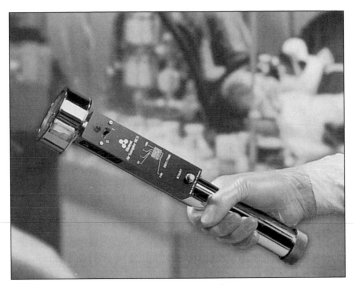

Fig. 8.1. Active sampler (Abinghurst Biotest Ltd).

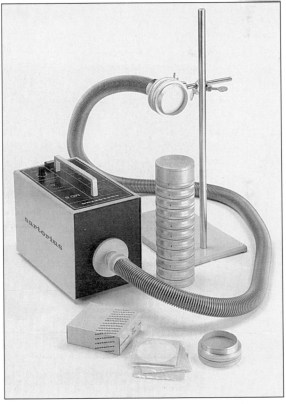

Fig. 8.2. Active sampler with cascade impacter (Sartorius Instruments Ltd).

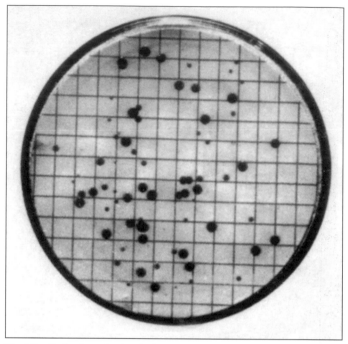

Fig. 8.3. Settle plate after incubation (Sartorius Instruments Ltd).

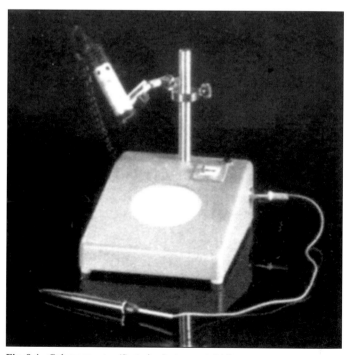

Fig. 8.4. Colony counter (Sartorius Instruments Ltd).

vicinity of the equipment that contains them; e.g. fermenters, centrifuges, filters and pipes in which they are processed to detect leakage of aerosols. Where possible a sample should be taken in these locations. An appreciation of air flow patterns must be established when sampling plans are drawn up, which may be useful in interpreting the results.

The measurement of contamination levels

Measurement of total particulates

Micro-organisms attach themselves to dust particles or liquid droplets. The two most common methods employed are:

Membrane filtration and microscopy

This consists of drawing a sample of air through a membrane filter for the measurement of total airborne dust as described in Chapter 1. A grid membrane filter is used with an appropriate sampling train and air flow rate. The trapped particles are counted using a microscope with an eyepiece micrometer. This method is time-consuming and requires skill and experience in examining the samples and interpreting the results correctly. It is therefore not a practicable method for routine monitoring of the workplace.

Optical particle counters

The sampled air is passed through a light-scattering device. The sampling rate is usually fixed and particle counts of different size ranges are displayed. White light is usually used for measurement of levels of particles drawn to 0.5 μm in size. A laser light is required if the particles are smaller.

With this technique the user needs to be aware of several shortcomings. Accurate counts of 0.1 μm particles are not reliable as the near-forward light-scattering instruments have a 'blind spot'. Furthermore, the instruments that have low sampling rates may not take a sufficiently large sample to enable the environment to be examined critically. Due to the dynamic range, greatly differing sized particles cannot be measured simultaneously. The length of the sampling tube needs to be considered to prevent larger particles greater than 5 μm falling out within the tube if the sampling tube is too long.

When monitoring for microbial levels the methods currently available are not automated nor can they be carried out remotely, in contrast to the methods for the measurement of dust, radiation or gases and vapours. Methods that measure metabolic activities of microbes and uptake of radioactive substances are being developed. The methods are therefore intrusive since the person undertaking the monitoring has to enter a critical area or disturb the operatives to take environmental samples. The data obtained may not therefore be representative of the conditions under which the critical process takes place. With the exception of settle plates and possibly the liquid impingement methods, the techniques do not allow continuous sampling throughout a work procedure.

Usually a combination of settle plates, air samples, surface samples and operatives' finger dabs are used because of the limitation of each individual method for the examination of critical environments.

Measurement of microbial levels

Active, passive and surface sampling methods are employed for the measurement of microbial levels. For passive sampling settle plates are commonly used. Several types of air sampler are available. Where plates are used, they are incubated and examined as for settle plates.

Measurement of airborne micro-organisms using settle plates

Aim
The aim is to estimate airborne micro-organisms using settle plates. It is a basic passive sampling technique used to evaluate the concentration of micro-organisms in workroom environments. The Petri dishes can contain selective or non-selective culture media.

Equipment required
For each location to be sampled simultaneously, the following are needed: a settle plate (usually 90 mm or 140 mm diameter), each poured with nutrient medium; an incubator; a microscope; and a facility for staining and identification of micro-organisms.

Method
1 Place the plates in appropriate sampling locations.
2 Remove lids and note time.
3 At the end of the sampling time cover plates and note the time.
4 Incubate under the conditions specified by the microbiologist and examine (by expert).
5 Record the number of colony-forming units (cfu) and types of micro-organisms.
6 If necessary identify the micro-organisms present.

Possible problems
1 Though this procedure is relatively cheap and easy to perform and involves few stages, the operator must have prior knowledge

of the background levels of micro-organisms and their preference for nutrient medium.

2   Sampling volume is not known.

3   The nutrient may dry out.

4   The variation of contamination levels throughout the sampling period cannot be seen.

Active sampling

Slit to agar sampler. This is designed to collect on culture media any organisms that are present in large volumes of air. The air sampled is drawn through slits and the micro-organisms impinge on rotating agar plates. The dimensions of the slits and the distance from slits to agar surface and the air flow are controlled to give maximum impingement. For example, the Casella sampler draws air at the rate of 700 l min^{-1} and the recommended sampling time is 5 minutes. The sampling time may be extended by coating the agar with hydrophilic wax. The plates are incubated and the numbers of colonies counted. As the volume of air sampled and the rate of rotation of the turntable are known, the viable count per litre of air can be calculated.

Single sieve sampler. The air sampled is drawn through slits and the particles impinge on a 55 mm agar plate. An example is the SAS sampler (see Table 8.2) in which the distance from the perforations to the agar surface is not as highly controlled as in the slit sampler, making this sampler less efficient at capturing airborne contaminants. The sampling volumes will be large enough to examine most critical environments but it can be cumbersome to use.

Cascade sampler. This is also known as a sieve sampler. The air sampled is drawn through perforations onto a stack of agar plates. Each agar plate is separated by perforated metal plates, the size of the perforations decreasing from the top to the bottom of the stack. Larger particles impact on the top agar plates and the smaller particles cascade over and through the perforations until they impact on the appropriate plate lower in the stack. An example is the Anderson sampler where the sampling rate is 3 l min^{-1}. This may be too low for the critical examination of work areas.

Centrifugal sampler. These are usually battery operated and so are hand-held, making them useful for fieldwork. The sampled air is drawn into the sampling head by means of an impeller that directs the air onto an agar strip fitted around the circumference of the sampling head. An example is the Biotest Folex sampler (Fig. 8.1) in which the sampling rate is 40 l min^{-1} based on a micro-organism size of 4 μm. The strip is incubated, the numbers of colonies counted and the viable count estimated. Strips containing selective and non-selective media are available. Since larger particles may also be captured, the sampling rate could be increased, but the interpretation of the data will be more difficult.

Liquid impingement. The air sampled is drawn through an aspirator bottle containing a suitable medium. This is used as the bubbler described in Chapter 1. After the specified sampling time the solution is filtered, plated, incubated and examined as described for settle plates.

Filtration. The air sampled is drawn through a membrane or gelatine filter. The filter is then plated out, incubated and examined.

Surface sampling

Work and other surfaces may become contaminated with microbes involuntarily deposited by employees or raw materials. They may therefore be direct or indirect sources of infection. Surface sampling is carried out using cotton swabs, contact plates or finger dabs.

Aim

The aim is to measure surface microbial levels. The initial stages of all three techniques are described before the material is transferred onto a growth medium.

Equipment required

For swabs: sterile cotton swabs, buffer solution, agar plates for each sampling spot.
For contact plates: 55 mm Rodac plates, with the agar poured to the brim to give a convex surface.
For finger dabs: agar plates.
For all: an incubator, a microscope, and a staining facility.

Method

For swabs:
1   Wet the cotton swab with buffer solution.
2   Draw the swab across the sample surface. An area of a flat surface can be sampled by making a template of a specified area, such as 100 cm^2, and wiping the area with the swab.
3   Roll the swab across the surface of an agar plate and cover with lid.

4 Alternatively, the fluid containing the microbes can be squeezed out of the swab into a known volume of liquid culture medium.

For contact plates:
5 Open a plate and place the convex agar against the surface to be sampled so that the agar is in contact with the surface to be sampled for 0.5–1 min. Cover with a lid.

For finger dabs:
6 Open a plate and ask an operative to touch the surface of an agar plate with the tips of all fingers and thumb.

For all methods:
7 Incubate (as directed by a microbiologist).
8 Examine and identify the micro-organisms.
9 Record the number of colony-forming units and types of micro-organisms present.

Analysis of data
Like other monitoring data analyses a statistical approach is recommended because of the imprecision of the methods and techniques, the low levels of contamination and the natural variability of the levels.

Acknowledgement
We wish to thank Sartorius Instruments Ltd for their advice on the handling of micro-organisms.

References and further reading
Advisory Committee on Dangerous Pathogens (1990) *Categorisation of Pathogens According to Hazard and Categories of Containment*. HMSO, London.
Advisory Committee on Genetic Manipulation (1988) *Guidelines for the Large Scale Use of Genetically Manipulated Organisms*. ACGM/HSE Guidance Note No. 6. HMSO, London.
Advisory Committee on Genetic Manipulation (1988) *Guidelines for the Categorization of Genetic Manipulation Experiments*. ACGM/HSE Guidance Note No. 7. HMSO, London.
Advisory Committee on Genetic Manipulation (1988) *Laboratory Containment Facilities for Genetic Manipulation*. ACGM/HSE Guidance Note No. 8. HMSO, London.
Advisory Committee on Genetic Manipulation (1989) *Guidance on the Genetic Manipulation Regulations*. HMSO, London.
Ager, B.P. and Tickner, J.A. (1985) *The Control of Micro-organisms Responsible for Legionnaires' Disease and Humidifier Fever*. Occupational Hygiene Monograph No. 14. Science Reviews, Leeds.
BSI Standards (1973) *Specification for Small Incinerators*. BS 3107. BSI Standards, Milton Keynes.

BSI Standards (1973) *Specification for Large Incinerators.* BS 3316. BSI Standards, Milton Keynes.

BSI Standards (1975) *Medical Specimen Containers for Microbiology.* BS 5213. BSI Standards, Milton Keynes.

BSI Standards (1976) *Environmental Cleanliness in Enclosed Spaces.* BS 5295. BSI Standards, Milton Keynes.

BSI Standards (1979) *Specification of Microbiological Safety Cabinets.* BS 5276. BSI Standards, Milton Keynes (revised 1989).

Brown, C., Campbell, I. & Priest, F.G. (1987) *Introduction to Biotechnology.* Blackwell Scientific Publications, Oxford.

Church, H.T.V. & Balus, K. (1988) *Safety in Higher Education and Research Establishments – a Guide to Safe Practices.*

Clark, R.P. (1983, 1989) *The Performance, Installation, Testing and Limitations of Microbiological Safety Cabinets.* Occupational Hygiene Monograph No. 9. Science Reviews, Leeds.

Collins, C.H. (ed.) (1985) *Safety in Biological Laboratories.* Institute of Biology, London and John Wiley, Chichester.

Collins, C.H. (1988) *Laboratory Acquired Infection: History, Incidence, Causes and Prevention,* 2nd edn. Butterworths, London.

Collins, C.H. (ed.) (1988) *Safety in Clinical and Biomedical Laboratories.* Chapman & Hall, London.

Collins, C.H. & Grange, J.M. (1990) *The Microbiological Hazards of Occupations.* Occupational Hygiene Monograph No. 17. Science Reviews and H & H Scientific Consultants, Leeds.

Collins, C.H. & Kennedy, D.A. (1987) Microbiological hazards of occupational needlestick and 'Sharps' injuries. *Journal of Applied Bacteriology,* **62**, 385–402.

Collins, C.H., Lyne, P.M. & Grange, J.R. (1989) *Collins and Lyne's Microbiological Methods,* 6th edn. Butterworths, London.

Cottam, A. (1988) *The Selection and Use of Disinfectants.* Health and Safety Executive Technology Division. Specialist Inspector Report No. 17. HMSO, London.

Department of Health and Social Security (1978) *Code of Practice for the Prevention of Infection in Clinical Laboratories and Postmortem Rooms.* HMSO, London.

Dixon, B. (1988) *Engineered Organisms in the Environment.* Society for Applied Bacteriology, Aberdeen.

Dunsmore, D.J. (1986) *Safety Measures for Use in Outbreaks of Communicable Disease.* WHO, Geneva.

Fromer, W. *et al.* (1989) Safe biotechnology III. Safety precautions for handling microorganisms of different risk classes. A Report of the Working Party on Safety in Biotechnology of the European Federation of Biotechnology. *Applied Biotechnology and Microbiology* **30**, 541–552.

Glass, D.C., Hall, A.J. & Harrington, J.M. (1989) *The Control of Substances Hazardous to Health: Guidance for the Initial Assessment in Hospitals.* Department of Health, HMSO, London.

Grist, N. & Emslie, J.A.N. (1985) Infections in British Clinical Laboratories 1982–3. *Journal of Clinical Pathology* **38**, 721–714.

Grist, N. & Emslie, J.A.N. (1989) Infections in British Clinical Laboratories 1984–5. *Journal of Clinical Pathology* **40**, 826–829.

Grist, N. & Emslie, J.A.N. (1989) Infections in British Clinical Laboratories 1986–7. *Journal of Clinical Pathology* **42**, 677–681.

Health and Safety Executive (1987) *Legionnaires' Disease.* Guidance Note No. EH/48. HMSO, London.

Health and Safety Executive (1989) *Consultative Document: The Control of Legionellosis – Proposals for Statutory Action.* CD18(F). HMSO, London.

Health and Safety Executive (1989) *Radiation Safety for Operators of Gamma Irradiation Plants.* UK Panel on Gamma and Electron Irradiation. HMSO, London.

Health Service Advisory Committee (1982) *The Safe Disposal of Clinical Waste.* HMSO, London.

Health Service Advisory Committee (1985) *Safety in Health Service Laboratories: Hepatitis B.* HMSO, London.

Health Service Advisory Committee (1986) *Safety in Health Service Laboratories: The Labelling, Transport and Reception of Specimens.* HMSO, London.

Kennedy, D.A. (1988) Needlestick injuries: mechanism and control. *Journal of Hospital Infection* **12**, 315–322.

Lieberman, D.F. & Gordon, J.G. (eds) (1989) *Biohazards: Management and Control.* Marcel Dekker, New York.

Microbiological Consultative Committee, Society for General Microbiology (1986) *Guidelines for Microbiological Safety,* 3rd edn. HMSO, London.

Organization for Economic Cooperation and Development (1986) *Recombinant DNA Safety Consideration.* OECD, Paris.

Royal Society of Chemistry (1989) *COSHH in Laboratories.* RSC, London.

Russell, M. (1990) *Principles of Biological Monitoring.* Tutorial No. 5, Parenteral Society, Cambridge.

Shanson, D.C. (1982) *Microbiology in Clinical Practice.* Butterworths, London.

Social Security (Industrial Injuries) (Prescribed Diseases) Regulations (1985) DHHS, London.

Sussman, M., Collins, C.H., Skinner, F.A. & Stewart-Tull, D.E. (eds) (1988) *The Release of Genetically-Engineered Micro-organisms.* Academic Press, London.

The Health and Safety (Dangerous Pathogens) Regulations (1981) HMSO, London.

The Reporting of Injuries, Disease and Dangerous Occurrence Regulations (RIDDOR) 1985 (1986) HMSO, London.

US Public Health Service (1988) *Centers for Disease Control/National Institute of Health Biosafety in Microbiological and Biomedical Laboratories,* 2nd edn. US Government Printing Office, Washington.

World Health Organization (1983) *Laboratory Biosafety Manual.* WHO, Geneva.

9 Surveys

Introduction

The main objectives of monitoring the exposure to health hazards of employees are to ensure that exposures are kept to a minimum and that any authorised limits are not exceeded.

The foregoing chapters have indicated the methods of taking workplace environmental measurements and the instruments available to do so but it is important to realise that to obtain a true picture of the health hazards of a working environment no single measurement will suffice. With regard to workplace pollution, it rarely occurs in a way which is evenly spread, in concentration or intensity, over the whole workplace or over the whole working period. In the case of the emission of a gas or particles of dust the concentration is greatest at the point of emission but it may fluctuate as the process progresses. As the pollutant moves away, its behaviour and dispersion will depend upon the air currents occurring in the room and therefore will vary with the movement of people, machinery, and both natural and mechanically induced air currents. Even one shift may not be typical of another in the same place due to the variability and cyclic nature of many processes. With regard to noise in the workplace, it is unlikely that levels will remain constant throughout the working period, and some employees move from one noisy workplace to another.

Surveys must be planned within the resources available to obtain the best possible information on the hazards as they affect individual employees and on the workforce as a whole. In general, the more measurements that are taken, over the longest period of time, the more reliable the results will be. If important decisions are to be made or expensive equipment purchased following the results of monitoring, then the measurements must be as accurate as possible, be scientifically valid, and be taken by a trained and competent individual.

The benefits that accrue from a well-designed and planned programme of monitoring include:

- An indication that engineering and containment standards are suitable and sufficient.

- The use of the data collected in various ways such as: risk-benefit analyses; medical-legal purposes; observation of trends; and epidemiological studies.

- The motivation of supervisors and employees to reduce exposure by increasing health and safety standards as a result of the information gained from monitoring.

- The identification of high levels of exposure that may occur during the malfunction of any procedures or processes.

- A demonstration that operations are carried out correctly.

Ideally a comprehensive monitoring programme should include the measurement, evaluation and recording of all exposures incurred by all employees involved in a discrete work activity. The methods used for monitoring that should be considered are: (1) personal monitoring, for airborne contaminants, which could be total/inhalable or respirable/alveolar; (2) workplace monitoring; (3) the measurement of contamination where necessary; and (4) biological monitoring. A system of monitoring must be able to:

- Specify the type and extent of monitoring that must be carried out.

- Select suitable instruments, dosimeters and analytical techniques.

- Test, calibrate and maintain equipment.

- Carry out monitoring and sample collection.

- Analyse, process and interpret monitoring data.

- Maintain monitoring records.

- Produce a system for reporting the monitoring results in an appropriate form to management, supervisors, employees and safety representatives and other interested parties.

- Check on reproducibility and quality assurance of monitoring techniques.

- Correlate monitoring data with medical and other observations made.

- Monitor implementation of recommendations resulting from monitoring results.

Planning

An assessment of the work process or activity will determine the measures required to control employees' exposure and the need to carry out routine monitoring of the workplace or monitoring at specified times.

It is important to plan any survey. A visit to the measuring sites should be made wherever possible before any monitoring is carried out. If the site is far too distant to make a visit then a plan of the areas to be surveyed should be obtained. These plans must show the position of the main emitters of pollutants, heat, noise or radiation together with the location of the operators.

A full complement of equipment is required at the site before starting. To have to return to base for some forgotten item is, at best, time wasting and, at worst, impossible. One or two days of measuring time can be lost when away from home-base if some vital item is missing. Check lists are given for survey items and are offered as a guide (Tables A9.1–A9.6, pp. 245–247). They should be supplemented if additional items are required and in the light of experience. It may not be necessary to include every item on every list but it is better to consider and reject rather than not to consider at all.

A photograph of the workplace is an invaluable aid to memory, particularly when it is inconvenient to return to the site. Therefore, a camera has been included in all check lists but permission must always be sought to use it. A video recording camera is also a useful adjunct to a survey particularly if a dust lamp is used, as the movement of dust around the nose of a worker or in front of a ventilation hood can be re-examined during the report-writing stage of the survey.

The check lists also contain items of protective clothing since the places where surveys are required may contain health hazards. Health and safety professionals need to protect themselves and set a good example to others.

Manpower

It is always useful to plan a survey involving two people, one of whom need not be involved in the technical aspects, but should be available to record results and note the workplace operations that are taking place. A single surveyor can easily become harassed if too much work is attempted and under such pressure vital information is not recorded and unrepeatable data are lost. A good surveyor will come with record sheets already prepared with columns for every item to be noted and as each reading is taken will note its value in the appropriate place. The amount of work that can be done in a shift will depend upon the layout of the work area to be surveyed but it is wise not to undertake too much. For example, in the case of an airborne dust survey, no person should be expected to have more than ten sampling pumps running simultaneously without the help of an assistant, and if the area to be covered involves several workrooms then even less than this should be planned.

The places where sampling is being carried out over a period of time should be supervised, not only to make a note of the type of activities that are being carried out, but to watch the equipment to minimise the risk of pilfering and to ensure that the results are not adversely affected by deliberate over- or under-exposure. It has been the authors' unfortunate experience occasionally to have a handful of dust thrown across a sampling filter or a charcoal tube placed above the surface of a solvent emitter in order to deliberately increase the concentration measured. The opposite sometimes occurs where the sampling device is placed in a fresh air situation to ensure that a low concentration is obtained. The continued presence of the surveyor will minimise the occurrence of such deliberate actions.

Calibration

The reliability with which monitoring measurements can be performed depends on the accurate calibration of instruments and their routine maintenance. This should be done by a competent individual according to the manufacturers' instructions.

Procedures for monitoring

Decisions must be made on the monitoring strategy. When and how the monitoring will be carried out should be specified and the measuring or sampling methods to be used must be determined. The locations and sampling frequency must be decided on and consideration must be given to how the results are to be interpreted and presented. For example, sampling may be carried out on a representative group only or may be carried out during periods when exposures are likely to be high.

To obtain the best estimate of exposure a structured approach is necessary. This should be based on knowledge and experience of the site. It may be helpful to carry out an initial appraisal of the area to be monitored; followed by a basic survey and then finally a more detailed survey. The results of these may indicate if some form of regular monitoring is required. Knowledge and experience of the site will also suggest the protective equipment required for the health and safety professional for the period of the monitoring.

The initial appraisal can serve the following purposes:

1   Indicate, identify or define the problem.
2   Show the range and pattern of exposure, highlighting the likely deviation of results.
3   Provide the order of magnitude of the exposures to compare with published or company standards.

From this information a more detailed survey can be planned with confidence. Alternatively, it could show that further measurement is unnecessary.

A procedural approach should suggest whether a full shift sample is necessary or whether sampling over a shorter period would be more appropriate. For example, an operative may work in an area for part of the shift where exposure is high but for the remaining time he or she may be in an area where exposure is low. A full shift sample will indicate the worker's *time-weighted average* exposure on that day but would not indicate how much of that exposure was obtained from the high-exposure source. On another day he may spend more time in the high area giving rise to a greater time-weighted average exposure. At times, spot samples or samples taken during the shift with natural gaps for meal breaks or rest periods may be more useful.

Workplace monitoring

Whenever possible personal monitoring should be carried out which, for airborne pollution, should be in the breathing zone of the worker, preferably as close to the nose as is socially acceptable. However, this is not always possible and environmental or 'static' monitoring may be the only recourse available. For example, it is unwise to ask a worker to carry a glass bubbler containing a liquid reagent as it may become broken or spilt. A static sampler placed as close to the worker as possible has to suffice but it may underestimate the true exposure.

Workplace monitoring usually measures airborne contamination and can be divided into either routine or operational monitoring.

Routine monitoring ascertains whether airborne concentrations are satisfactory for continuing operations. It is a confirmatory activity but may include provision for the detection of the onset of abnormal or emergency conditions.

Operational monitoring supplies information about a particular operation, procedure or workplace. It is useful where routine monitoring is not feasible or when specific procedures are carried out.

Special monitoring is carried out for various reasons such as to check the adequacy of control equipment; to examine an operation that is carried out under abnormal conditions; to confirm design specifications; to settle disputes; or to investigate certain features. Special monitoring is therefore of limited duration with clear objectives and is terminated once the problems are identified or decisions taken on the appropriate routine or operational monitoring.

The selection of employees to be sampled poses certain problems if representative exposure data are required for a group of people who undertake substantially the same work and are exposed to the same substance(s). There is a choice between selecting those with the maximum exposure or randomly selecting employees within a group. If the maximum-exposure group is required a well-informed judgement is needed to ascertain who falls within that group. This needs an intimate knowledge of the work process and the way the job is being undertaken. For a health and safety professional coming into the plant with little knowledge of the process it is better to select those to be sampled randomly. Various authorities give advice on how to choose, recommending minimum numbers based upon the total size of the workforce employed on that process. For example, NIOSH suggest that out of a group of eight employees seven should be selected; out of a group of 15, 12 should be selected; and out of a group of 50, 18. This presupposes that all the chosen employees will agree to be sampled and that sufficient sampling equipment and personnel are available to cover the load.

Whenever a survey is to be undertaken that involves worker cooperation it is important to make contact with the employees' representative and to explain in some detail the purpose of the survey, what is required from the workforce and who will receive the results. It may be necessary to demonstrate to them the equipment to be used and how it is positioned. This may have to be done several days before the survey to allow for feedback and to allay any apprehensions.

Results

Standard records sheets should be drawn up, which must contain the following information:

• the location of the sample to include reference to a sketch plan or photograph of the workplace;

• whether the sample was personal, that is taken in the breathing zone of a worker, or static, that is close to the workplace but in a fixed position;

• if static, how close it is to the source of pollution, noise or radiation;

• if personal, the employees' names and job being undertaken;

• the results of the measurement: airborne concentration, noise level or dose, radiation level or dose;

• the date, time and duration of the sampling period;

• details of any special conditions prevailing at the time that may make the results untypical;

• whether personal protective equipment was being worn during the sampling period and, if so, the type.

The results should only be quoted to three significant figures unless it can be demonstrated that the degree of precision is greater. For example, it would be unwise to quote an airborne concentration of a substance to more than 1 decimal place if in mg m^{-3} or to the nearest unit if in parts per million, whilst with decibels a round number would suffice for type 2 meters and no more than one decimal place for type 1 meters.

It is not within the remit of this book to give advice on the interpretation of results, but standards have been referred to under the various operations where applicable. Standards for workplace environments are published by various sources, some of which are listed in the further reading section, but it must be remembered that standards are offered as a guide and not as the strict dividing line between what is hazardous and what is not. Action should be recommended to improve the situation if levels of more than 25% of the recommended standard are observed, as these indicate a rising trend or that conditions are approaching that standard. Also, there may be persons present in the workplace who are more susceptible to the pollutant than those for whom the standard was chosen.

When all the results of a particular survey are available it is advisable to examine them carefully to ensure that they are representative of the workplace. Every possible confounding factor should be considered and places and times when errors could have occurred in the measuring technique should be noted. Above all, it is important to bear in mind that monitoring results can, at best, only give an estimate of the environmental hazards present and it is unwise to stick rigidly to the occupational exposure standard (OES) or other criteria and standards.

Records of monitoring

Recently it has become a legal requirement to keep records of monitoring results. For example, the Codes of Practice associated with the Ionising Radiation Regulations, Control of Substances Hazardous to Health, Noise at Work Regulations, etc., lay down record-keeping requirements. The national requirements influence the purpose of record keeping and the nature and scope of the records that are kept. They may involve demonstration of compliance with regulations, evaluation of trends of exposure, collective monitoring results, individual monitoring results for legal or medical purposes, study of effects in exposed population, or the demonstration of good housekeeping standards.

The system of record keeping must be such that records can be easily retrieved and interpreted at a later date, perhaps many years later. Also, factory inspectors may require to see them to establish compliance.

It is advisable to record as much detail as possible on the exact location of particular employees and the type of work that was being carried out at the time of monitoring. This must include:

• Quick, easy and unambiguous identification of employees.

• Details of the place of employment and type of work and activities carried out when the monitoring was undertaken.

- Where the sampling locations were situated.
- What procedures were used, including specification of equipment, duration of monitoring, and operations during monitoring.
- Recording of observations in a form that is readily retrievable and understood, and that can be easily correlated with the corresponding health records.

Records of workplace monitoring are important because they should be able to provide evidence that satisfactory working conditions have been maintained and where necessary indicate trends in workplace concentration so that adverse health effects can be prevented. Systematic monitoring information has greater significance for long-term records. Records obtained from isolated monitoring serve to guide employees in the control and improvement of prevalent working practices.

Monitoring records are usually made available to:

- the individual worker;
- the employer;
- the regulatory authority; and
- insurance and other related organisations.

Further reading

American Conference of Government Industrial Hygienists. *Threshold Limit Values for Chemical Substances and Physical Agents in the Workroom Environment*. ACGIH, Cincinnati, published annually.

Brown, R.R. (1995) The sampling of gases and vapours. In: *Occupational Hygiene* (eds J.M. Harrington & K. Gardiner), pp. 84–98. Blackwell Science, Oxford.

Dewell, P. (1989) *Some Applications of Statistics in Occupational Hygiene*. HH Scientific Consultants & Science Reviews, Leeds.

Gardiner, K. (1995) Sampling strategies. In: *Occupational Hygiene* (eds J.M. Harrington & K. Gardiner), pp. 287–307. Blackwell Science, Oxford.

Health and Safety Executive. *Occupational Exposure Limits*, Guidance note EH40. HSE Books, Sudbury, Suffolk, published annually.

Health and Safety Executive (1997) *Monitoring Strategies for Toxic Substances*, Guidance HS(G) 173. HSE Books, Sudbury, Suffolk.

International Labour Office (1977) Occupational Exposure Limits for Airborne Toxic Substances. ILO, Geneva.

Jones, A.L., Hutcheson, D.M.W. & Dymott, S.M. (1981) Planning surveys and use of results. In: *Occupational Hygiene, an Introductory Guide* (eds A.L. Jones, D.M.W. Hutcheson & S.M. Dymott), pp. 151–157. Croom Helm, London.

Mark, D. (1995) The sampling of aerosols. In: *Occupational Hygiene* (eds J.M. Harrington & K. Gardiner), pp. 99–122. Blackwell Science, Oxford.

National Institute of Occupational Safety and Health (1977) *Occupational Exposure Sampling Strategy Manual, 1977*. US Department of Health, Education and Welfare, Cincinnati.

Oakes, D. (1995) Statistics. In: *Occupational Hygiene* (eds J.M. Harrington & K. Gardiner), pp. 324–349. Blackwell Science, Oxford.

Appendix

Table A9.1. Dust survey equipment check list

Item as required	Amount	Packed	Returned
Adhesive tape			
Camera and film			
Carrying case			
Clip board			
Cyclone filter holder			
Dust lamp			
Electronic calculator			
Filters (weighed)			
Filter holders and covers			
Forceps or tweezers			
Harnesses			
Knife			
Labels			
Membrane filters			
Paper			
Pens and pencils			
Petri slides			
Petri dishes			
Plastic bags			
Pumps – high flow			
Pumps – medium flow			
Results sheets			
Rotameter and calibration chart			
Safety pins			
Scissors			
Screwdrivers (small)			
Smoke tube kit			
String			
Tape measure			
Tripods			

(*continued*)

Table A9.1. (*cont.*)

Item as required	Amount	Packed	Returned
Tubing			
Timer or stop watch			
Safety clothing:			
shoes			
goggles			
helmet			
respirator			
gloves			
overalls			
ear defenders			

Table A9.2. Gases and vapours survey equipment check list

Item as required	Amount	Packed	Returned
Adhesive tape			
Adsorbent tubes			
Bubblers (empty)			
Bubblers (full)			
Bubbler reagent			
Camera and film			
Carrying case			
Clip board			
Colorimetric detector tubes and pump			
Direct reading instrument			
Electronic calculator			
Filters			
Filter holders			
Forceps or tweezers			
Harnesses			
Knife			
Labels			
Passive samplers			
Paper			
Pens and pencils			
Plastic bags			
Pumps – low flow			
Pumps – medium flow			
Result sheets			
Rotameter and calibration chart			
Safety pins			
Sampling bags: mylar or tedlar			
Scissors			
Screwdriver (small)			
Smoke tube kit			
String			
Tape measure			

(continued)

Table A9.2. (*cont.*)

Item as required	Amount	Packed	Returned
Tripods			
Tubing (check bore)			
Vacuum tubes			
Timer or stop watch			
Safety clothing:			
shoes			
goggles			
helmet			
respirator			
gloves			
overalls			
ear defenders			

Table A9.3. Thermal survey equipment list

Item as required	Amount	Packed	Returned
Adhesive tape			
Aspirated psychrometer			
Botsball thermometer			
Camera and film			
Carrying case			
Clip board			
Distilled water			
Dry bulb thermometers			
Electronic calculator			
Globe thermometer (large) and charts			
Globe thermometer (small) and charts			
Heat index charts			
Kata thermometer and charts			
Natural wet bulb thermometer: wicks and beakers			
Paper			
Pens and pencils			
Psychrometric charts			
Reflective foil and corks			
Results sheets			
Sling psychrometer (whirling hygrometer)			
Smoke tube kit			
Spare thermometers			
Spare wicks			
Tape measure			
Thermos flask and hot water			
Timer or stop watch			
Tripod:			
stand			
boss heads			
clamps			

(*continued*)

Table A9.3. (*cont.*)

Item as required	Amount	Packed	Returned
WBGT meter			
Safety clothing:			
shoes			
goggles			
helmet			
respirator			
gloves			
overalls			
ear defenders			

Table A9.4. Ventilation survey equipment check list

Item as required	Amount	Packed	Returned
Anemometer, heated head type			
Anemometer, vane type			
Aneroid barometer			
Camera and film			
Calibration charts			
Carrying case			
Clip board			
Desk fan			
Diaphragm pressure gauge			
Drill and bit for hole boring in ducts			
Electronic calculator			
Log–linear graph paper			
Manometers			
Manometer liquid			
Marker pen			
Paper			
Pen and pencils			
Pitot-static tubes			
Plasticine or 'Blu-tack'			
Plugs for holes in ducts			
Results sheets			
Smoke tube kit			
Tape measure			
Thermometer			
Timer or stop-watch			
Tracer gas			
Tracer gas detector			
Tubing for gauges and manometers, blue and red			
Safety clothing:			
shoes			
goggles			
helmet			

(*continued*)

Table A9.4. (*cont.*)

Item as required	Amount	Packed	Returned
respirator			
gloves			
overalls			
ear defenders			

Table A9.5. Noise survey equipment check lists

Item as required	Amount	Packed	Returned
Batteries, spare for meters			
Calibrator			
Camera and film			
Carrying case			
Clip board			
Dosimeters			
Electronic calculator			
Microphones for meters			
Microphone extensions for meters			
Noise rating curves			
Octave band analyser			
Octave band charts			
Paper			
Pens and pencils			
Pistonphone			
Results sheets			
Screwdriver (small)			
Sound level meters			
Tape measure			
Tape recorder, connections and tapes			
Tripods			
Timer or watch			
Safety clothing:			
shoes			
goggles			
helmet			
respirator			
gloves			
overalls			
ear defenders			

Table A9.6. Lighting survey equipment check list

Item as required	Amount	Packed	Returned
Calibration charts			
Camera and film			
Carrying case			
Clip board			
Daylight factor meter			
Electronic calculator			
Graph paper			
Hagner Universal Photometer			
CIBSE Code			
Measuring tape (10 m)			
Munsel charts			
Paper			
Pens and pencils			
Photometer			
Results tables and plans			
Screwdriver (small)			
Tape measure			
Safety clothing:			
shoes			
goggles			
helmet			
respirator			
gloves			
overalls			
ear defenders			

10 Assessment of risks to health

Introduction

To manage health and safety successfully in any work area the serious and frequent health risks need to be identified, and preventative or control measures must be put in place to protect employees from the risks. Occupational illness, accidents and near misses can highlight weakness and provide an opportunity to put things right. However, it is better to be proactive and take an organised approach to make sure that illness at work, accidents and near misses do not occur in the first place.

There are several steps in managing health and safety in the work place – the first is to have a health and safety policy. This should outline who has responsibilities for health and safety, how the hazards are identified and risks assessed and what is the procedure to control the risks. It is essential to organise the work staff to ensure that they have the competency to carry out their work safely. This will require a training needs analysis to identify any extra instruction or training requirements, appointing relevant people with particular health and safety duties such as risk assessment co-ordinators, radiation protection supervisors, etc., and making sure that they have the skills and resources to carry them out. Arrangements may have to be made for specialists to undertake specific activities such as testing and examining pressure systems, testing water for micro-organisms etc. if these are not available in-house. It may be necessary to consult employees on work processes and develop practical or realistic solutions to problems and informing employees about the risks involved in their work and the precautions they need to take. All this needs careful planning. Systems must be put in place to measure performance both before and after things go wrong. This can be done by auditing against the workplace standards that have been set and ensuring that improvements identified in risk assessments have been put in place. All illnesses, accidents and near misses should be reported and investigated. All this will indicate where further improvements can be made, and assessment of health risks is part of this.

All the above is enshrined in the various health and safety regulations that have arisen out of the UK Health and Safety at Work (Etc.) Act 1974 and European Health and Safety Directives. The further reading list at the end of this chapter shows most of the relevant UK legislation and associated guidance and should help where assessments are required in specific areas.

Assessment of risks to health are usually carried out in a health and safety risk assessment. Risk assessments can be qualitative or quantitative. When qualitative techniques are used the risk is expressed in levels such as high, medium or low and are based on judgement and not on numerical calculations. Quantitative methods express risk in numerical terms and are based on calculations. At the planning stage of plant design these can be complex and specialists are usually employed to carry them out.

A qualitative approach is often sufficient to assess health risks but it may be necessary to obtain some simple quantitative data. This can be obtained by measuring exposure through monitoring, as described in the preceding chapters. For chemicals this could be the measurement of exposure to dusts, gases, vapours or the efficacy of ventilation systems. For physical conditions the measurement of heat, noise or lighting levels may need to be measured and related to operatives' exposure.

These measurements need to be interpreted in terms of risk. Therefore, health risk assessments use both quantitative and qualitative approaches.

The Management of Health and Safety at Work Regulations require that all hazards and risks are identified and controlled from a given activity. The most effective way to do this is to identify the need for a health risk assessment as part of an integrated risk assessment. When hazards are identified, relevant specific assessment such as Control of Substances Hazardous to Health (COSHH), noise and Display Screen Equipment (DSE) may have already been carried out. These should be reviewed and, if still valid, should be cross-referenced to the health risk assessment.

Purpose of risk assessment

A health and safety risk assessment is a systematic identification of the hazards associated with an activity and the evaluation of the risks associated with those hazards. An employer's duty to safeguard the health and safety extends not only to his employees but also to anyone else who could be adversely affected by the activities of a particular job. This will include contractors, visitors and members of the public.

To prevent occupational injury, ill health, disease, and property damage, various systems are used to identify the causes of failures in management control, which can cause harm or damage. These can be proactive or reactive. An example of a reactive system is accident reporting and investigation. An example of a proactive system is risk assessment. When a risk assessment is undertaken the events or activities that could cause harm are identified and the associated risk is evaluated; the likelihood or probability of their occurring and the severity of the associated consequences. With information on the level of risk presented by the activities of the workplace, decisions can be made on the best way to control the risk.

Risk assessment is the first stage in controlling injury and ill health in a workplace. It is not just a paper exercise or a compliance issue. The conclusions of the risk assessment must be acted upon and continuously monitored for effectiveness. Risk assessment is part of risk management of a workplace to minimise risks and improve the health and safety of employees. Risk management encompasses other activities such as plant design, emergency plans, safe operating instructions, training, auditing and monitoring performance indicators.

The stages of a risk assessment

Look for the hazards

List all the activities undertaken in a particular area. Identify the hazards associated with each activity that are routinely and non-routinely performed. Note the environmental aspects and examine the workplace layout and process. Hazards that are reasonably fore-seeable should be noted and decisions taken on their significance. The insignificant risks should be noted to indicate that they have been considered but the significant ones will require more attention.

Decide who might be affected and how

Make a list of all personnel who may be exposed to the hazards, including how many people and who they are. It is usual to identify work groups or type of employees such as process workers, maintainers, welders, office workers, etc., and also non-employees such as contractors, customers, neighbours, etc. Estimate the harm that could be realised, which includes acute or chronic effects, minor or major injury, etc.

Evaluate the risks arising from the hazards and decide whether existing precautions are adequate or more should be done.

The issues that need to be addressed here will cover:

- the method of work;

- the circumstances and deviations from normal procedure;

- the frequency of operation;

- whether it is a routine task;

- whether the legal requirements that are specific to the activity are being satisfied.

For complex processes job safety analysis may be required to tease out the risks and hazards.

The risks are then quantified and several techniques can be applied at this stage.

Examine the control measures

Consider and define the preventative and/or control measures that could reduce the risk: measures to reduce or control risks to health and safety are given later in this chapter.

Once the control measures have been assessed, any further measures that are deemed to be required must be listed. This may require a cost benefit analysis and the various jobs may have to be prioritised.

Once the controls are installed they need to be monitored and maintained. This includes:

Monitoring against standards.

Maintenance procedures, both planned and breakdown.

Cleaning schedules.

Testing and examination of specified parts of equipment or plant.

Environmental monitoring.

Health surveillance.

Auditing and inspections.

Record the significant findings

Risk assessment should be recorded if 5 or more people are employed in a workplace: an example of a record form is shown in Annex 10.1.

Review the assessment regularly and revise it if necessary.

In certain cases risk assessment must be reviewed at specified intervals. Risk assessments must be revised when circumstances change. Examples of this include when a work method changes, when a substance is changed, new equipment is introduced, the level of activity changes, etc. This will ensure a continued safe working environment.

Benefits of health risk assessment

The main benefit of a health risk assessment is the protection of employees, as the implementation of appropriate control measures will lead to a reduction in occupational accidents and ill health. It also provides the means for resources to be prioritised with a programme to meet targets. This gives the opportunity to spread the resources in time and money over a reasonable period of time. Risk assessment can be used to rationalise activities and processes as it will provide the opportunity to look carefully at how the activities are undertaken and may highlight potential savings if something is changed for the better. It can also help in making management decisions on major investment. However, it must be appreciated that there are uncertainties at every step in a risk assessment as predictions are made on what might happen. This makes it an inexact science.

As can be seen, risk assessment serves a variety of purposes, an important one of which is compliance with legislation. In particular, compliance with regulation 3 of the Management of Health and Safety in the Workplace Regulations and the safety policy duty as required under the Health and Safety at Work (Etc.) Act 1974. Risk assessments are an important part of management tools that help to ensure that the health and safety policy is effective. They also provide easily updated records that clearly show the justification for the health and safety arrangements.

Hazard and risk

The definition of risk assessment terms vary. Table 10.1 gives the definitions given in various HSE publications.

Table 10.1. Definitions of hazard and risk

Source	Definition of risk
COSHH, 1988	risk from a substance as being 'the likelihood that it will harm anyone in the actual circumstances of use'
Successful Health and Safety Management	'the likelihood that a specified undesired event will occur due to the realisation of a hazard by, or during, work activities or by the products and services created by work activities'
The ACOP for MHSWR	'the likelihood that the harm from a particular hazard is realised'

Source	Definition of hazard
COSHH, 1988	'potential to cause harm' (this harm could be damage to skin, organs, bones etc. with adverse effects on breathing, circulation, hearing or offspring)
Successful Health and Safety Management	'potential to cause harm' (including ill health and injury)
The ACOP for MHSWR	'something with potential to cause harm'

A hazard is something that has the potential of something to cause harm, e.g. chemicals, energy, machines, etc. Risk is the chance, which can be in a range from large to small, of that harm actually occurring to a particular target. Hazard and risk can be expressed in words, numbers or any other way, as long they are meaningful. If there is no target then there is no risk.

The severity of harm is the quantity of a substance to which an operative is exposed and the length of time of exposure. The time of exposure will depend on the activities undertaken and can be obtained by observation or asking the operative to record their times spent on each of the activities carried out. As described in preceding chapters this can be overcome by using time-weighted averages.

For substances hazardous to health such as dusts, gases, vapours or micro-organisms the chance of exposure is determined by the level of containment of the material and the route of entry into body, which could be by inhalation, ingestion, injection, or skin absorption by contact.

Care should be taken to ensure that possible accidental exposures by inhalation are considered. These include spillages, activities such as cleaning and maintenance that can disturb deposited material thereby making them airborne again, entry into confined spaces that contain hazardous substances, and wearing contaminated clothing as personal protective clothing. Rules that prohibit eating, drinking, smoking, applying cosmetics, nail biting etc. prevent substances hazardous to health entering the body by ingestion.

Risk is hazard multiplied by potential of exposure

Risk/Assessment is a quantitative or qualitative evaluation of the chance that a hazard will cause harm.

This will identify and consider all the significant factors that can affect the probability and extent of harm and will assist management in deciding whether such circumstances need to be eliminated or improved to decrease the chance. Only then can decisions be made on the most effective control measures.

Legal requirements

Risk assessment has been required by health and safety legislation for some time now. The purpose is to encourage employers to have systems for assessing, monitoring and controlling risks of their operations. Risk assessment is implicit in the Health and Safety Work (Etc.) Act 1974, which brought health and safety controls into all areas of work. The concept of reasonable practicability was introduced, which implies the need for employers to assess risk to persons affected by their work and to provide a degree of control commensurate with the level of risk. The Management of Health and Safety at Work Regulations 1992 takes this concept one stage further by explicitly requiring employers to carry out a risk assessment. Other legislation that requires risk assessments is given in

Table 10.2. Clearly there will be a cost to industry in implementing this requirement but the cost could be recovered if it achieved a reduction in accidents or occupational ill health.

Table 10.2. The legislation that specifically requires risk assessment

Regulations	Hazard or risk to be assessed
Management of Health and Safety at Work Regulations, 1992	Risk to health and safety to employees, self-employed and third parties as a result of the work undertaken
Manual Handling Operations Regulations, 1992	Risk to injury from manual handling operations
Personal Protective Equipment at Work Regulations, 1992	Suitability of personal protective equipment
Health and Safety (Display Screen Equipment) Regulations, 1992	Risk to health and safety to users and operators in consequence of using workstations
Noise at Work Regulations, 1989	Exposure to noise
Control of Substances Hazardous to Health Regulations, 1988 and 1994	Risks to health from exposure to substances hazardous to health
Control of Asbestos at Work Regulations, 1987	Exposure to asbestos
Ionizing Radiations Regulations, 1985	Nature and magnitude of radiation hazard
Control of Lead at Work Regulations, 1980	Nature and degree of exposure to lead

The health hazards not covered by specific assessment legislation should be assessed under the MHSWR.

There is other legislation in which specialist risk assessments are required. These are listed in Table 10.3.

Table 10.3. Regulations that require specialist risk assessments

The Control of Industrial Major Hazard Regulations, 1984 as amended by the Control of Industrial Major Hazard (Amendment) Regulations, 1990

The Offshore Installations (Safety Case) Regulations, 1992

The Railways (Safety Case) Regulations, 1994

The Genetically Modified Organisms (Contained Use) Regulations, 1992

The Management of Health and Safety at Work Regulations require a 'suitable and sufficient' risk assessment. Risk Assessment is an on-going procedure that requires regular review and, where necessary, revision. It is not a one-off job that is filed and forgotten once carried out: it must be sustainable. In some legislation the need to review is specified usually when new substances, equipment or people are introduced into the existing system or when alterations are made to procedures, processes or premises. Revisions are necessary when monitoring procedures indicate that the current control measures are not working effectively. A suitable and sufficient risk assessment will reflect what employees are reasonably expected to know about the hazards associated with their undertaking.

Who should carry out risk assessment

Some regulations specify that 'competent' persons carry out the risk assessment, for example the COSHH Regulations. The HSE's definition of a 'competent person' is someone who has 'the necessary experience, knowledge, training and instruction to do the job competently'. This implies that the competent person has the ability to recognise their own limitations.

The Management at Work Regulations does not specify that 'competent persons' should carry out the risk assessment, although competent persons are required to implement and monitor the control measures identified by the assessment. It therefore implies that competent persons are required to be involved in undertaking the risk assessment.

In practice, persons who carry out the assessments will depend on the risks identified and the resources available. This may involve assistance from in-company or external advisors, experts or consultants. Usually, larger companies have specialists such as safety professionals, occupational hygienists and engineers to assist; smaller organisations use in-house expertise of work processes.

Enforcement action with regard to risk assessment

Risk assessments were originally a specialist field confined to high-hazard industries such as the chemical and nuclear organisations, but they are now required in the majority of workplaces and are fundamental to the successful management of occupational health and safety. When risks in a workplace are not demonstrably trivial and assessments are not carried out, then the employer may be issued with an enforcement action from an enforcing authority if there is a breach of criminal law. The level of enforcement action, which could result in an improvement or prohibition notice and ultimately prosecution under criminal law. This will depend on the circumstances. The employer could also be open to a civil case if it can be shown that a duty of care is breached.

Risk assessments also identify the relevant statutory requirements relating to the activities undertaken. If these are not identified then the corresponding control measures may not be implemented or procedures followed as may be required by the legislation. This could happen whether or not this leads to an accident.

The content of risk assessment

Risk assessment is part of a comprehensive health and safety management system and not an isolated procedure. Smaller companies may not have a high degree of sophistication but nevertheless there is normally a safety management system in place. The success of the safety management system of a work area will depend on the accuracy and thoroughness of its risk assessments.

The risk assessment should be suitable and sufficient and should identify significant risks. It should identify and prioritise control measures appropriate to the nature of the undertaking. Therefore, the risk assessment for a small, simple organisation with relatively few hazards may be a straightforward exercise based on experience and judgement with little need for specialised skills or techniques. However, in larger more complex organisations 'quantified' risk assessment may be required. Clearly the detail contained in a risk assessment is directly related to the risk. The Approved Code of Practice accompanying the Management at Work Regulations indicates that it is not necessary to itemise every trivial hazard. The exceptions are where the hazard may be influenced by other factors, which then make it significant and where risks, which are not reasonably foreseeable, would not be expected to be anticipated beyond the limits of current knowledge. The Approved Code of practice also recognises that it will not be necessary to repeat a risk assessment for comparable hazards in situations that are static, i.e., where there are no changes. In dynamic situations where there are frequent changes to the work or workplace or where mobile or visiting employees are present, such as in the construction industry, the risk assessment may define a broad range of likely risks and rely on detailed planning and employee training to take account of and control the risks as and when they arise.

Risk assessment in practice

As mentioned above a variety of disciplines are usually involved in the risk assessments to cover all aspects of an activity. A typical risk assessment would involve making use of the operators undertaking the task, along with safety, environmental, medical and engineering professionals. Other specialists may also be invited to participate.

Identification of hazards

Risks cannot be effectively controlled unless it is known what they are. Therefore the first stage of a risk assessment is to identify the risks and to assess them.

Before the risk assessment can begin some relevant information must be collated on the following:

- Activities undertaken
- Equipment used
- Materials and substances involved
- Procedures employed
- Work area involved
- Personnel present all or part of the time, during the duration of the activity.

From this, a further list should be made of anything that can cause harm together with details of the harm that can be caused. This will include risks in all areas of work, in all the work activities undertaken, with all the products handled and services undertaken. Different approaches may be required to suit particular situations. Risk assessments can be carried out for groups of hazards, e.g., access, workplaces, substances, machinery, process equipment, electrical equipment, etc. It may be more appropriate to look at hazards inherent in the operations e.g. production, maintenance, office tasks, packing, dispatch, warehousing, etc. Whatever approach is taken the risk assessment should be aimed at improving the health and safety standards in the workplace.

Assessment

It is necessary to check if specific risk assessments have been carried out to satisfy the requirements of other legislation such as COSHH or PPE. These can be used in the overall risk assessment with appropriate cross-referencing and need not be repeated although they should be reviewed to ensure their validity.

All risks must be assessed and the findings recorded. Accord each risk a rating on the basis of the scale used (see Table 10.4) and decide on a particular cut-off point after which a risk is considered to be trivial. This allows account to be taken of the legal requirements as well as the aims set out in the safety policy. There is debate about ignoring trivial risks to avoid excessive paperwork and it is believed that it will result in more important risks being obscured. However, it is more thorough, effective and efficient to record all risks related to the work activity.

Separate the trivial risks from the rest and keep a record of them. Trivial risks are risks arising from routine activities associated with life in general that can be ignored unless the work activity compounds those risks or there is evidence of significant relevance to the particular work activity. Focus on risks that are liable to arise because of the work undertaken.

Assessment of risk rating

A risk rating for each hazard is obtained by multiplying a probable frequency rating by a severity rating. Table 10.4 gives an example of the scales. Descriptions used to define the numbers vary as does the range of numbers. Croners recommend that there should be a minimum of three and a maximum of eight. A higher number should always represent a greater probable frequency and greater severity.

Table 10.4. Example of scales

	Probable frequency		Severity
1	Improbable occurrence	1	Trivial injuries
2	Possible occurrence	2	Minor injuries
3	Occasional occurrence	3	Major injury to one person
4	Frequent occurrence	4	Major injuries to several people
5	Regular occurrence	5	Death of one person
6	Common occurrence	6	Multiple deaths

Some assessors prefer to use more than two scales. For example, the severity scale can be split into two – one representing the nature of possible harm from an unwanted event (harm severity) and the other representing the number of people who could be harmed (scope severity).

The individual ratings will be a matter of judgement and foresight based on knowledge and experience. Once the individual ratings are agreed upon, the risk rating for each hazard is calculated.

An example is given to illustrate this using figures taken from Table 10.4:

1   A regular occurrence would have a probable frequency rating of 5, and if it could cause a major injury to one person it would have a severity rating of 3 giving a risk rating of 15 (3×5).

2   An occasional occurrence would have a probable frequency rating of 3, and if it could cause major injuries to several people it would have a severity rating of 4 giving a risk rating of 12 (3×4).

The hazard rating of 15 is higher than 12 so before considering other factors it is rated as a higher priority for control.

Assessment for risk control rating

Examine each hazard with regard to factors that may increase the risk rating for some or all groups and factors in relation to the control measures that are already in place which decrease the risk rating. These factors must be identified and described and the individual ratings reassessed using the scales to calculate a new risk rating. The risk level must be reduced to as low as is reasonably practicable (ALARP).

Identification of control measures

Make decisions on whether existing control measures are adequate and what improvements or additions can be made, taking into account the relevant legislation and in-house standards. Where the need for additional or improved measures are identified these findings must be used to amend the health and safety policy, and arrangements for planning, implementing, controlling and monitoring the safety measures. Ways in which some common risks that can be reduced or controlled in a variety of workplaces are given in this chapter.

Existing controls need to be reviewed as part of health and safety risk assessment to evaluate the chance of exposure. In particular circumstances measurements need to be taken: for example, checking the effectiveness of exhaust ventilation systems. Some of these measurements could be legal requirements such as testing and examination of extraction systems under COSHH Regulations. If the controls are not engineering controls they are safe systems of work; these need to be checked to be sure the risk is adequately controlled.

Prioritising

It is important to prioritise the improvements required, as everything cannot be done at once for a variety of reasons. High-risk situations should be tackled first. An action plan should then be prepared indicating what will be done when. The sequence could follow:

1   Identify the problems using the risk assessment.
2   Consider the possible solutions to the problems, which may involve using a multidisciplinary team.
3   Select the best solution.
4   Make detailed plans on how to implement the improvements.
5   Organise the resources needed in terms of time, people and money.
6   Carry out the improvements.
7   Check the effectiveness of the improvements and assess if further improvements are required.
8   Review the system.
Note: The statements 4, 5 and 8 involve prioritising the improvements.

Records

All risk assessments must be recorded to show clearly how the assessments were carried out and the conclusions reached. Examples of record forms are given in Annexes 10.1 to 10.7.

It is important to appreciate the purpose of risk assessment. It is to determine the control measures necessary to prevent or at least protect against the risks to health and safety in the assessment.

Once the risk assessment is complete, appropriate control standards and objectives need to be set and the control measures necessary to achieve them identified. Systems should be in place to monitor the control measures implemented to ensure their effectiveness and efficiency in achieving the control standards. Also, review procedures need to be incorporated.

The following gives a summary of the risk assessment procedure:

1   Consider all tasks and situations.
2   Identify all the hazards that are or may be involved (people, material, equipment, environment).
3   Identify those who may be exposed to the hazards.
4   Analyse the risks of injury, ill health or loss from the hazards.
5   Evaluate whether the risk is adequately controlled.
6   Consider measures that may eliminate or reduce risk further in line with the basic principles of hazard control.
7   Implement the risk control measures.
8   Monitor the measures.
9   Review and feedback any corrective action.
10   Record assessment, taking into account new control measures.

Assessment of exposure and control measures

After the risk assessment is complete consideration needs to be given to the way in which improvements can be made or ways in which the risk can be reduced. The following gives some of the most frequent risks that are identified in assessments and strategies for reducing the risk. It can be seen that monitoring for health hazards is part of health risk management. Once the control measures for improvements have been put in place it is best to monitor them to ensure that the chance of injury from the relating operations have been reduced and assess if more improvements can be added.

To assess exposure to hazardous substances to health

An example of a recording form is given in Annex 10.2.

The COSHH Regulations are the main regulations for controlling workplace exposure to substances that are hazardous to health (ionising radiation, asbestos and lead have their own regulations). COSHH requires employers to:

1   Assess risks to health arising from exposure to hazardous substances.
2   Prevent or adequately control exposure.

3   Ensure control measures are used, maintained, examined and tested.

4   In some instances monitor exposure and carry out appropriate health surveillance.

5   Inform, instruct and train employees.

Substances hazardous to health are gases and vapours (see Chapter 2), liquids and solids that may be in the form of dust, powders granules etc. (see Chapter 1). There are labelled as very toxic, toxic, corrosive, harmful or irritant. They are also micro-organisms (see Chapter 8), dusts, fumes and other materials that can impair the health of employees. The effect on the employee will usually depend on how hazardous the substance is, and the level and length of time of exposure. For many airborne substances such as dusts, gases and vapours that may be inhaled, exposure limits have been set that should not normally be exceeded.

Hazardous substances could be the raw materials, intermediate products of the process of manufacture, by-products, finished products or waste products. Employees may be affected by various routes of exposure by the:

- inhalation of airborne particles, gases or vapours,

- ingestion of solids, dusts and liquids,

- skin contact with solids, dusts and liquids. Some substances that may pass through the skin can result in systemic impairment while others may injure the skin resulting in possible dermatitis.

Pre-assessment procedures

In undertaking a COSHH Assessment it will be necessary to undertake some pre-assessment procedures in order to gather the necessary information. These are discussed below.

1   Decide on the extent of the area to be assessed. This will be governed by the likely size of the final assessment documentation. For example, a complete production process may involve several workstations and many chemicals, which would make the final documentation unwieldy. In this case it might be better to break the process up into activities, each having their own assessment.

2   List the substances present in the chosen activity.

3   Note the quantities of the substances involved and the type of containers in which they are housed.

4   Determine which of those substances are actually used. For example, some substances not used in the activity may still be stored in the area. These should be safely disposed of or stored elsewhere.

5   Find out their true chemical names and CAS (Chemical Abstracts Series) number. Note: every chemical is issued with this unique number that positively identifies it. Use of this number is always advised, particularly when chemicals have long complicated names and a slight misspelling may refer to another substance. They can be found in the 'approved supply list' issued under the Chemicals (Hazard Information and Packaging for Supply) Regulations 1994 (CHIP), and are also shown in EH40.

6   Obtain manufacturers' materials safety data sheets.

7   Evaluate these data sheets as they may understate the true hazardous nature of the substance. It may be necessary to consult a toxicological reference book to verify the information given.

8   Produce a new data sheet to suit the conditions pertaining in the workplace under assessment. The manufacturer's data sheet, however accurate, will not be written in the company's own house style, nor will it reflect the way the substance is being handled in the place being assessed. Furthermore, the data provided may be too technical to suit the education and experience of the personnel handling the substance and in some cases may not be written in the language of the operators. Many industrial employees may not be sufficiently fluent in the language of the country in which they work to be able to understand the information they are being given to safeguard their own health.

9   Determine the mode of exposure, e.g. inhalation or skin contact and decide whether airborne concentrations require measurement. If they do, arrange for surveys to be undertaken.

Once these preliminary tasks have been undertaken, the assessment can proceed. The record form shown in Annex 10.2 will act as a guide to the procedure and will form the final record.

To reduce and control of risks from substances hazardous to health

If the assessment shows that the substance(s) need to be controlled in better ways than they are then advice is given in the COSHH Code of Practice (1994).

These paragraphs show a hierarchy of controls that can be followed to either prevent risk of exposure or to control it.

It will be necessary to consider in the order given whether:

1   the hazardous substance can be eliminated altogether, e.g. by changing the processes or the product specification;

2   the hazardous substance can be replaced by a less hazardous material with the same properties or in a less hazardous form, e.g. dusty granules that can be replaced by pellets or liquids;

3   the exposure to the hazardous material can be reduced by engineering controls such as: total enclosure, partial enclosure with local exhaust ventilation (LEV) (see Chapter 4);

4   whether total automation of the process can be applied thus reducing the time people are exposed to the hazardous material;

5   whether the exposure time can be reduced in some other way.

Check if personal protective equipment (PPE) is required. Normally this should be applied in addition to the above measures but, if required, the standard recommended must give protection against the hazards. Ensure that the user knows how to use the equipment correctly, that it fits properly, and that it is cleaned, maintained and stored according to the manufacturer's instructions so that it is always efficient and fit to use. Although it is better to control exposure by engineering methods, the use of PPE is frequently the only temporary solution.

If the substance is identified as a carcinogen then COSHH puts great emphasis on the need to control and includes all of the above.

Decide what control measures or improvements can be applied, then put them in place and monitor them to check if they are effective. This can be done by measurement of airborne concentrations in the breathing zone of the operators as described in Chapters 1 and 2. With ventilation equipment this has to be done at regular intervals in accordance with COSHH Regulations, and by means of measurement techniques described in Chapter 4.

The risks can be reduced by:

1   Identifying all the hazardous materials used for all work operations. Valuable information can be obtained from suppliers' data (e.g. labels and safety/hazard data sheets), the knowledge on the work site, previous experience, guidance from the HSE, trade associations and industry contacts.

2   Assessing what risks are present for the way in which each substance is handled. Consider how an exposure might occur, the people that may be affected and the control measures that are already in place.

Note: the most hazardous material may not have the greatest risk. For example, a highly toxic material handled in a totally enclosed system for the whole process will have a low risk, but a mild acid or alkali handled with inadequate precautions may lead to irritation and possibly dermatitis. As this could also affect a large number of employees it is a potentially higher risk.

3   Not exceeding the occupational exposure limit (MEL, OES, 'Asbestos Control Limit' or 'Lead in Air Standard') if a hazardous substance has one (these are listed in the current EH40).

4   Checking to see what else can be done to reduce the risk further.

Health surveillance

Setting up programmes to undertake health checks can identify if employees are affected by the tasks they undertake at work. In some instances specific health checks are required by the legislation e.g. work with lead, vinyl chloride monomer etc.

Further steps that can be taken include:

• If there are any known risks in the operations undertaken inform the employees of them and the precautions that must be taken.

• Take note of the complaints that indicate similarities.

• Carry out trend analyses of the accident and illness data to pinpoint problem areas.

• Encourage employees to report ill health problems, and provide medical care.

• Encourage employees to tell their doctor about their occupations and the materials handled with the safety data sheets.

To assess risk of exposure to heat and cold

Four parameters are measured and taken into account together when assessing exposure to heat (see Chapter 3). They are:

• the temperature of working environment, the 'dry bulb temperature';

• the amount of moisture in the working environment, the 'wet bulb temperature';

• the air velocity in the working environment;

• the radiant heat exchange between the skin of the operator and the surroundings.

A single index, the WBGT, brings the wet and dry bulb and globe temperatures together to represent the exposure to heat from which the risk to health can be calculated.

To reduce and control risk from heat stress

This will depend on the dominant condition; the following measures could be applied:

• shield the operative from a radiant heat source if possible;

• reduce the air temperature;

• slow down work rates;

• increase the air velocity;

- build breaks into the work programme or have a work/rest regime. The rest periods include work in cooler environments, to reduce exposure time;

- ensure that appropriate clothing is worn;

- encourage operatives to participate in physical fitness programmes;

- discourage operatives who are obese or have a history of cardio-vascular problems to work in areas where there is a possibility of risk.

To assess exposure to cold or hypothermia

Two parameters are measured:

- dry bulb temperature;
- wind velocity.

The heat loss from the body is calculated using charts (see Chapter 3). The wind chill index is the most important.

If the operative is wet or sweats, the rate of body heat loss is increased, and if the wind speed increases the body heat loss increases further even if the air temperature remains the same.

To reduce risk from hypothermia

- Wear several layers of appropriate clothing with the outer garment made of windproof material.

- Introduce work/rest regimes in which the rest breaks are taken in the warm.

- Increase the rate of work.

To assess exposure to noise

There are many noisy processes carried out in workplaces that have the potential to damage hearing, e.g. milling, grinding, bottling etc. Regular exposure to high noise levels can cause short-term or irreversible deafness (see Chapter 5). The longer an employee is exposed and the higher the noise level the greater the damage to hearing.

Identify the operators who might be exposed to noise above the first action level or peak action and areas where noise may be a problem.

Measure room noise levels and personal noise levels if appropriate (see Chapter 5).

To reduce exposure from noise

1 Develop an action plan to reduce exposure to the noise. This can be achieved by controlling the noise at source. Wearing ear protection should be the last resort.

2 Where possible, eliminate the source of the noise.

3 Select quiet machines or processes when looking at production or other operational methods.

4 Apply anti-vibration damping or change the frequency of vibration.

5 Where possible, put noisy machines in separate rooms.

6 Change the acoustic properties of the room and shield the noisiest machines.

7 Enclose noisy machines and processes with sound-proofing materials.

8 Organise the work and 'rest periods' so that employees are in the noisy areas for the minimum amount of time.

9 Reduce the duration of exposure by job rotation or by providing a noise refuge such as an acoustically treated control room.

10 Where hearing protection is provided, ensure that employees are given the appropriate information and training to ensure that they are being used correctly.

11 Monitor that improvements have reduced the noise exposure to the level specified.

12 Assess to see if further improvements can be made.

To assess exposure to vibration
See Chapter 5.

To reduce of risk from vibration

• Get the best grip, push used to guide and apply the tool – the tighter the grip the more vibration energy is transferred to the hand.

• Reduce the exposure pattern by changing the length and frequency of work and rest periods.

• Reduce the amount of hand exposure to vibration.

• Ensure good blood circulation by ensuring that working temperature is acceptable for the duration of the activity.

• Encourage a healthier lifestyle, which includes no smoking and frequent exercise, to allow good blood flow through the body.

To assess risks associated with micro-organisms or biological agents

Guidance for work with specialist biological agents, especially in research work, is given in the Advisory Committee on Dangerous Pathogens Categorisation of biological agents according to hazard and categories of contaminant. Usually a qualified Biological Safety Officer will co-ordinate these assessments of health risks. The following factors need consideration for the possibility of infection.

- The hazard groups. This will include:
    the size and nature of the activity;
    the control measures already in existence and their effectiveness;
    the possible and infective dose;
    the immune status of the operatives;
    the susceptibility of outsiders;
    the route of infection;

- The routes of infection along with the virulence and transmissibility of the organisms;

- The work and the likely release of infectious material both in routine work and accidents;

- The quantity of material handled during the activities;

- Reduce and control of risks from micro-organisms or biological agents;

- The work undertaken in the appropriate contaminant.

The risks associated with some common biological agents:

Legionellosis. The risk of this could affect all employees. The HSE guidance on the prevention and control of Legionellosis (including legionnaires' disease) should be consulted.

Hepatitis B and HIV. These are a possibility after a needlestick injury if a sufficient volume of contaminated body fluid is transmitted. Procedures must be in place to prevent puncture of the skin with contaminated materials.

Clinical waste. Health care staff, transporters and incinerator operators would be at risk from harm in relation to clinical waste. Guidance can be obtained from the appropriate authorities regarding the safe disposal of clinical waste.

Zoonoses. When animals and birds and their products are handled, the possible occupational zoonotic diseases should be considered.

The risk from an individual zoonotic disease will depend on the current incidence rates. Some, such as anthrax and bruccllosis, have almost been eradicated in the UK but Weils' disease or Leptospirosis and psittacosis and chlamydia infections can be of concern.

The following are some of the issues that arise from health risk assessment, which also need to be controlled or reduced.

To assess exposure to manual handling

Many operations require handling loads of various weights and shapes. This requires lifting, carrying and moving loads, which could result in injury usually in the neck, shoulders, back, legs and arms. If a load is heavy or if incorrect handling techniques are used then just a few manoeuvres can result in an injury. Working with lighter loads in a repetitive manner can also result in cumulative damage over a period of time, often known as work related upper limb disorder (WRULD).

To assess exposure to manual handling:

• identify the activities that involve manual handling;

• identify the risk of injury in each activity;

• assess if it is practicable to automate or mechanise the operations;

• undertake risk assessment and record findings (see Annex 10.3 for record form). Video filming the manual handling could help to analyse the activity and get a better understanding of the operations.

To reduce risk from manual handling operations

To reduce the risk from manual handling operations a risk assessment should be carried out in which the tasks where injuries are likely to occur must be identified and decisions must be taken on the most appropriate actions. This may involve changing how the task is carried out or improving the manual handling techniques. This will involve what the employee does, how the job is done and the best way to achieve it. This could include:

• Eliminating the task where possible.

• Reorganising the task to eliminate or reduce manual handling aspects. This can be achieved by automating or mechanising the task to remove or reduce the manual handling operations.

• Minimising the amount of manual handling by using lifting or other mechanical aids.

• Introducing materials that have to be manually handled in packages that can be handled easily.

- Planning breaks in the task or including job rotation to avoid long periods of repetitive work.

- Training relevant employees in good handling techniques.

To assess risk to work-related upper limb disorder (WRULD)
The services of an ergonomist may be required for this, who should:

- Identify specific activities.

- Estimate the degree to which they may affect the likelihood of injury by looking at the task and the design of the equipment, which includes movements, posture, the duration of activity, and the forces applied.

- Review organisational factors such as management activities and operator involvement, work organisation, training of the operator, or bonus systems.

- Review operator factors, including size in relation to equipment operator anxiety, and operator's external activities.

- Review workplace environmental factors such as noise, protective clothing, lighting and temperature.

To assess risk in workplace access and egress
Employees should have a safe access and egress to and from the work place. Accidents that can be possible from the risk assessment could be categorised as slips, trips, falls and those involving transport in the workplace.

Spilt materials can make floors slippery especially if they are on regular walkways and steps. Walkways with little grip also increase the chance of slips.

Trips are most often caused by poor housekeeping. Examples include walkways being obstructed, cables or pipes routed across walkways, poorly maintained access routes etc.

Falls occur most often when appropriate provision is not made for access to heights. A fall from a modest height can lead to serious injury if equipment or chemicals are involved.

Accidents with work vehicles such as forklift trucks, lorries and vans moving materials in workplaces is a possibility. Such accidents involve employees being struck or run over by moving vehicles, falling from vehicles, being struck by objects falling from vehicles or the vehicle overturning.

To reduce the risk from workplace slips, trips, falls and accidents with transport vehicles the chance of these occurring should be identified in the risk assessment then find ways of reducing the chance.

To reduce risk of slips:

• Use anti-slip footwear and finish floor surfaces with anti-slip materials.

• Design or modify equipment that handles fluids to prevent leaks and spillage.

• Use effective housekeeping procedures for spillage clean-up. Adopt methods of working and procedures that prevent spillage.

To reduce risk of trips:

• Allow no obstructions on access routes.

• Mark frequently used walkways to ensure that they are kept clear.

• Route pipes and cables away from walkways.

• Ensure that walkways are well maintained and repaired at the first sign of wear and tear.

• Design or modify access routes with care, e.g. doors and steps in appropriate places, handrails where necessary etc.

• Position equipment so that there is adequate room around it for the intended access.

To reduce risk of falls:

• Examine the frequency of the operations undertaken. If frequent access is required at a height, design or modify the equipment so that there is a permanent work platform. If access is required rarely, portable ladders, scaffolds or mobile elevating platforms can be used. If physical work activities need to be carried out platforms should be used in preference to ladders.

• Fit secure guardrails to any open edges, which are 2 or more metres in height.

• Fit guards to sharp surfaces or dangerous machines where the risk of injury is increased.

• Put in a system that ensures that all ladders, steps, handrails and work platforms are always in a safe condition.

To assess risk with work equipment
A variety of work equipment is used and each requires proper precautions to be taken. Injuries can occur in many different ways, some of which include:

• being entangled on rotating parts of equipment;

- being trapped between moving parts of equipment;

- being struck by moving equipment or parts of it;

- being struck by material ejected from the equipment;

- being trapped between moving equipment or parts and buildings or other fixed objects;

- being burnt from hot parts of equipment being used.

Different groups working on the machines may be affected in different ways. These include operators of the equipment, the people working near the equipment, maintenance and repair workers who may be contractors, or visitors to the work area. The risks arise during operations such as setting up, operating or cleaning the equipment and undertaking maintenance and repairs on the equipment.

To reduce risks from work equipment
1   Ensure that the equipment is suitable for the work to be carried out and it will withstand the conditions in which the work is carried out.
2   Prevent access to dangerous parts of the equipment. This can be achieved by enclosing the dangerous parts of the machinery with suitable fixed guards, interlocked guards or trip systems that use photoelectric devices, pressure-sensitive mats or automatic guards.
3   Ensure that the guards are kept in good working order.
4   Train operators in the safe use of equipment.
5   Ensure that temporary or inexperienced staff are always properly supervised.
6   Use safe procedures for non-operational work such as cleaning, repairing and maintaining. This may require the use of isolation systems or permit to work systems.

To reduce accidents with workplace vehicles
1   Ensure that the routes of vehicles are apart from the ones that are used by pedestrians.
2   Ensure that the routes for the vehicles are wide enough and well maintained.
3   Ensure that there are safe means of access on and off the vehicles.
4   Ensure a good maintenance programme for the vehicles.
5   Ensure that drivers carry out basic safety checks before using them.
6   Set up training programmes to ensure that the drivers carry out their work in a safe and responsible manner.

Electrical hazards

Most work areas need a supply of electricity to operate. The supply and equipment for electricity must be installed and maintained like other work equipment. There are many hazards associated with electricity, which include fire resulting from faulty installations, or contact with live parts which can cause burns and shock and in extreme cases death. Under special circumstances fire or explosions can be caused by electrical equipment or static electricity igniting flammable dusts, gases, vapours or mists. All electrical systems such as fixed equipment, portable equipment, wiring installations, battery sets, standby or other generators should be built to current standards and properly maintained to prevent any accident from occurring.

It is helpful to train users to carry out visual checks for signs of damage before the portable and transportable electrical equipment is used. This will include looking for the following:

• damage to the casing, cable sheath and plug;

• any exposed wires;

• imperfect joints in the cable that may be taped over;

• whether all the parts are properly secured to each other;

• evidence of the equipment being overheated, which shows up as discoloration or burn marks;

• if there is contamination with dirt or chemicals on it.

To reduce the risk from electrical hazards

1   Ensure that anyone working as an electrician has the relevant training and experience.
2   Ensure that all electrical equipment is of an appropriate design and built for the work it is required to do, checking that it is correct for the environment in which it is located. The plugs, sockets and switches must be appropriate and if the equipment is in a potentially flammable atmosphere it must be of the current explosion protected standard.
3   Have a good routine and breakdown maintenance programme for all equipment with records of inspections, tests and maintenance work carried out.

To reduce risk from fire

As people from high-risk categories such as the very old and young are involved, casualties from fire are higher in domestic premises than in workplaces. However, a significant number of employees are killed or injured each year due to fire in the workplace. For fire to break out the following are required:

- A source of fuel such as flammable gases, liquids or solids or combustible materials.

- A supply of oxygen: present in the air and additional sources can arise from oxidising agents.

- An ignition source, which could be hot surfaces, electrical equipment, static electricity, lighted cigarettes or naked flames.

It is more usual to concentrate on preventing a fire from starting but consideration must be given to minimising the consequences of a fire by installing fire detection and control systems such as fire and smoke detectors and alarms. In some instances, automatic water sprinklers are used. These reduce the rate at which the fire can spread so that the work area can be evacuated and the emergency services have time to arrive. It important therefore that an emergency procedure is in place and that employees are trained to respond in the correct manner.

To reduce the risk of fire from fuel

- Ensure good housekeeping is maintained so that combustible packaging and waste is kept to a minimum.

- Limit the quantities of combustible material in high-risk areas such as production by only holding enough for a shift or other suitable period.

- Store combustible material in separate areas or buildings and separate stocks of combustible materials by appropriate separation distances.

- Increase awareness of fuel sources such as flammable gases, liquids or solids and combustible materials, which are usually paper, card or other packing material.

- Encourage the use of non-flammable materials or materials with low flammability.

- Store flammable materials in a segregated area in safe containers or fire-resistant bins or cupboards.

- Ensure that there is adequate bunding or other suitable methods to contain spillage of flammable liquids.

- Design plant to stop flammable liquids and gases leaking by using remotely operated shut-off valves.

To reduce the risk of fire from oxygen

- Increase awareness of oxidising agents and keep them away from fuel sources.

- Segregate combustible materials from oxidising materials.

- Ensure that the workplaces are designed and built to resist fire with fire-stopped doors, roof spaces etc.

- Ensure that fire-extinguishing media such as water and foam carbon dioxide are available. The correct media must be available for the type of fire that might occur.

To reduce the risk of fire from ignition sources
Increase awareness of ignition sources and apply appropriate control measures where possible.

To reduce risks from explosions
Explosions have a great potential to cause injury, damage equipment and ruin buildings as they produce a rapid release of energy, which could result in exposure to harmful substances, and building collapse with flying debris. Fire could also be the result of explosions, especially when flammable materials are present.

Dust explosions
Dust explosions could occur when dusts from combustible solids are dispersed in air. This forms a flammable dust cloud, which could be set on fire and explode on contact with a source of ignition. The severity of the explosion will depend on several factors, which include the ratio of dust to air in the dust cloud, the confinement of the dust cloud and the type dust in the cloud. There are lower explosive limits (LEL) below which insufficient dust is present for the cloud to catch fire. However, one feature of dust explosions is that a small initial explosion, which could be initiated due to a gas or vapour ignition, could disturb dust that has collected in the work area especially on upper surfaces. This may add to the original dust cloud and could result in a bigger and more violent explosion.

Many processes such grinding and milling produce dusts, so the work equipment or plant can create explosible dusts inside equipment, which could get hot and start a fire. Ways to reduce dust cloud formation in machinery can be achieved by prevention of dusts within a process, dust leaking from equipment, fitting local exhaust ventilation on hoppers to prevent dust accumulation, or preventing dust leaking from containers such as sacks and bags. Good clean-down procedures will prevent the build-up of dust. Building design and layout is equally important with features such as locating equipment in open-sided buildings or away from the general employees and fitting relief vents so that equipment can vent to a safe place.

To reduce the risk from dust explosions

1 Ensure that the thermal stability information for the substances handled is known.

2 Eliminate substances and processes that could create flammable dust clouds where possible.

3 Substitute combustible substances or the material in a different form such as liquids and paste instead of powder.

4 Use de-dusting agents where possible.

5 Use good quality raw materials and prevent contaminating materials entering the equipment.

6 Design equipment that minimises the production of unwanted dust or overheating problems, and remove potential ignition sources.

7 Use local exhaust ventilation to remove unwanted dust clouds as they are formed.

To reduce the risk from pressure system explosions

When pressure equipment such as steam boilers, reaction vessels, pipes, air receivers and containers fail they burst or explode. Pressure equipment can fail for various reasons, such as the process going out of control, the equipment not being properly designed or built to withstand the temperature or pressure, the use of unsuitable materials, safety devices being missing or unsuitable, the equipment not being properly maintained. To minimise risks of injury it is best to:

• Site pressure systems away from the general workforce.

• Vent pressure relief valves and bursting discs to a safe area.

• Institute emergency procedures.

To reduce the risk from pressure system explosions, ensure that:

• the design and construction of the equipment is suitable for the process;

• the necessary safety devices such as pressure relief valves, bursting discs and emergency shutdown systems are in place and working properly;

• the monitoring systems are in place and functioning properly;

• the operating procedures are well written so that they are understood;

• operators are competent to do the job;

• equipment is properly maintained;

• emergency procedures and systems are in place and working.

To reduce the risk from flammable or explosive atmospheres containing gases, vapour, mists, or combustible dusts explosion
Explosions can occur in these atmospheres from ignition sources from electrical equipment and static electricity. The Electrical equipment is covered by the Equipment and Protective Systems Intended for Use in Potentially Explosive Atmospheres Regulations (ATEX) 1996 which places duties on suppliers and manufacturers to indicate CE marking and show which equipment group the appliance belongs to. Until 2003 appliances with the relevant BS/BS EN standard or other equally effective standard will be acceptable to the HSE.

Where atmospheres contain flammable/explosive vapours in which electrical equipment needs to be installed the areas should be classified into hazardous zones. British Standard 5345 provides guidance on selecting, installing and maintaining explosion protected electrical equipment. The zones are:

Zone 0: in which explosive gas/air mixture is continuously present.

Zone 1: in which an explosive gas/air mixture is likely to occur in normal operations.

Zone 2: in which an explosive gas/air mixture is not likely to occur in normal operation. If it does it will exist only for a short time.

To reduce the risk of the flammable/explosive atmosphere being ignited it is necessary to ensure that any electrical equipment used, fixed and portable, in a hazardous zone is constructed to a suitable explosion protection standard.

Dusts do not behave in the same way as gases and there is no current standard for zoning of explosive atmospheres of combustible dust clouds. The temperature of the hot surfaces needs to be monitored as the dust may ignite. Ingress of dust into electrical enclosures can cause problems as it may block ventilation holes or interfere with the cooling of electrical equipment. BS 6467 gives guidance on the design selection, installation and maintenance of equipment for use in the presence of combustible dusts. It is also good practice to locate electrical equipment away from the dust-producing work areas. BS EN 60529 gives guidance on the classification of electrical equipment enclosures according to the protection they give against hazards such as ingress of dust, water etc.

To reduce the risk of the combustible dust being ignited it is necessary to ensure that any electrical equipment used, fixed and portable, in a hazardous zone should be CE Marked or up to the BS EN standard.

The movement of certain liquids in actions such as pumping, filling or emptying vessels and powders can sometimes create a build-up of static electricity, which can cause a spark when discharged.

To reduce the static build-up

1   All conducting parts, especially metals, must be adequately earthed.
2   All equipment must be must be electrically bonded together and properly earthed.
3   Earth continuity must be checked regularly.
4   All earthing contacts must be kept clean and well maintained.
5   All portable containers should be earthed and connected to the fixed earthed equipment.
6   Use anti-static additives where possible.

Records

The appendices that follow are the authors' suggestions for keeping records of the assessments made. They can also be used as checklists to give guidance on the procedures to follow when making assessments.

Annex 10.1. Risk assessment/review record

1. **Risk assessor/co-ordinator**		**Assessment team**	
Name	Position	Name	Position

2. **Work activity/process**	
Building	Location
Description of activity/process	

Work is routine/non-routine
Frequency of work .... times per week/month/year/other

3. **Supporting documentation and references**	
COSHH assessment	PPE assessment
RPE assessment	Manual handling assessment
Method statement	Work authorisation form
Permit to work	Noise assessment
Other	

4. Risk assessment

Identified hazard	Groups affected	Severity	Probability	Risk level before controls	Existing controls	Risk level with control	Additional controls required	Action and date

5. Assessment reference

6. Date of assessment

Signatures	**Date**

Annex 10.2. COSHH assessment/review record

1. COSHH assessor/co-ordinator		Assessment team	
Name	Position	Name	Position

2. Work activity/process	
Building	Location

Description of activity/process

Work is routine/non-routine
Frequency of work .... times per week/month/year/other

3. Substances involved	MEL/OES	State	Quantity	Classification

4. Exposure				
Is there a chance of exposure?			yes	no
If yes, indicate level		high	medium	low
No. of people who may be exposed			directly	indirectly
Duration of exposure hours		Frequency of exposure times per day		

Other comments

5. Health risk	
Significant	Insignificant

(*continued p.280*)

Annex 10.2. (*cont.*)

6. Control measures	Type	Adequacy
Total enclosure		
Partial enclosure		
Local exhaust ventilation		
General ventilation		
RPE		
PPE		
Administrative		
None		
Other and comment		

7.   Assessment of control measures and recommendations/action required

8. Monitoring	Type	Adequacy
Health surveillance		
Exposure monitoring		
Comment		

9. Information, instruction and training	Type	Adequacy
Operating instructions		
Safe systems of work		
Safety data sheets		
Labelling		
Training		
Emergency procedures		
Comment		

10.   Review date

(*continued*)

Annex 10.2. (*cont.*)

11.   Signatures and dates
12.   Notes
13.   Supporting documentation references
14.   Assessment reference
15.   Date of assessment

Annex 10.3. Manual handling operations risk assessment/review record

1. Risk assessor/co-ordinator		Assessment team	
Name	Position	Name	Position
2. Work activity/process			
Building		Location	
Description of activity/process Work is routine/non-routine Frequency of work .... times per week/month/year/other Personnel involved			
3. Assessment			
Does the activity involve a significant risk of injury?			
If no, record this and the assessment is complete.			
If yes, how can the level of risk be reduced? Record results.			
Has the risk of injury been eliminated if it can be mechanised?			
Has the risk reduced to an acceptable level?			
If yes, record this and the assessment is complete.			
4. Checklist			

Does the task involve:	yes/no	comment
Holding the load away from the body?		
Twisting movements?		
Unnatural posture (stretching, bending)?		
Pushing or pulling that may cause strain?		
Lifting or lowering movements?		
Repetitive movements?		
Carrying loads to distances?		
Insufficient time for body to recover?		
A fast work rate?		
Other		

(continued)

Annex 10.3. (*cont.*)

5. Workload		
Is the work load:		
Too heavy?		
Difficult to hold?		
Bulky or awkward to hold?		
Unstable as the contents will move?		
Probably harmful (hot, cold, sharp, dirty)?		
Appropriately packaged?		
Other		
6. The environment		
Does the work area:		
Put constraints on body posture?		
Have uneven flooring?		
Include various levels of working?		
Have extremes of temperature, humidity?		
Have insufficient light?		
Have high noise levels?		
Have excessive air movements?		
7. Operators		
Does the handling require excessive strength?		
Does the handling require special information?		
Has the operator any health problems?		
Is the operator pregnant?		
Other		
8. Protective clothing		
Does the PPE increase the risk?		
Does the PPE decrease the risk?		
9. Overall risk of injury		
nil/low/medium/high		

(*continued p.284*)

Annex 10.3. (*cont.*)

10. Remedial actions	Completion dates

11. Assessment reference

12. Date of assessment

Signatures	Date

Annex 10.4. Display screen equipment risk assessment/review record

1. Risk assessor/co-ordinator		Assessment team	
Name	Position	Name	Position

2. Work activity/process

Building	Location

Description of activity/process

Work is routine/non-routine
Frequency of work .... times per week/month/year/other
Personnel involved

3. Assessment

Risk Factor	yes/no	action required
Display Screen		
Are the characters well defined and easy to read?		
Is the image free of flicker and movements?		
Is the brightness appropriate for the user?		
Is the contrast appropriate for the user?		
Does the screen tilt and swivel easily?		
Is the screen free from glare and reflections?		
Other		
Keyboard		
Can the keyboard be tilted?		
Is the keying position comfortable?		
Can the hands be rested comfortably at the keyboard?		
Is the keyboard free from glare?		
Are the characters well defined and easy to read?		
Other		

(continued p.286)

Annex 10.4. (*cont.*)

Furniture		
Is the work surface large enough for the equipment?		
Is the work top free from glare and reflections?		
Is there a document holder?		
Is the chair stable and adjusted to suit the user?		
Is there a foot rest?		
Is the user comfortable and free to move?		
Other		
Environment		
Is the working space sufficient for all movements?		
Is the air quality acceptable?		
Are physical conditions (heat, light, noise) acceptable?		
Other		
Software		
Is the user comfortable with the software?		
Other		
4. Assessment reference		
5. Date of assessment		
Signatures **Date**		

Annex 10.5. Noise risk assessment/review record

1. Risk assessor/co-ordinator		Assessment team	
Name	Position	Name	Position

2. Work activity/process	
Building	Location

Description of activity/process

Work is routine/non-routine
Frequency of work .... times per week/month/year/other
Personnel involved

3.   Assessment

Number of persons exposed	Noise level (L_{eq} or sound level)	Daily exposure period	$L_{ep,d}$ dB(A)	Peak pressure	Comments

4.   General comments

5.   Instruments used and date of last calibration

6.   Date of assessment

Signatures	Date

Annex 10.6. Personal protective equipment (PPE) assessment record

<table>
<tr><td colspan="2">1. Risk assessor/co-ordinator</td><td colspan="2">Assessment team</td></tr>
<tr><td>Name</td><td>Position</td><td>Name</td><td>Position</td></tr>
<tr><td></td><td></td><td></td><td></td></tr>
<tr><td></td><td></td><td></td><td></td></tr>
<tr><td></td><td></td><td></td><td></td></tr>
<tr><td></td><td></td><td></td><td></td></tr>
</table>

2. Work activity/process	
Related documentation	
Building	Location

Description of activity/process

Work is routine/non-routine
Frequency of work .... times per week/month/year/other
Personnel involved

3. Assessment

Duration of job

Physical effort required to carry out the job	high	medium	low
Are extreme temperatures likely to be met?	yes	no	
If yes, state	high	low	
Mobility required	normal	abnormal	
Visibility required	normal	abnormal	
Communication required	yes	no	
If yes, specify communication system required			

(continued)

Annex 10.6. (*cont.*)

Part of the body	At risk (tick)	Hazards	Degree of risk (low/medium/high)	PPE selection
Top of head				
Ears				
Eyes				
Respiratory system				
Face				
Whole head				
Hands				
Arms				
Feet				
Legs				
Skin				
Torso				
Whole body				

Confirmation that all items of PPE selected are adequate and suitable for the job

Confirmation that all items of PPE selected are compatible with each other

Confirmation that all items of PPE selected are acceptable to the wearer

Training required for the PPE selected?   yes   no

If yes, signature to confirm that adequate training has been carried out

Signed   Date

4.   General comments

5.   Date of assessment

Signatures   **Date**

Annex 10.7. Respiratory protective equipment (RPE) assessment record

1. Risk assessor/co-ordinator		Assessment team	
Name	Position	Name	Position

2. Work activity/process	
Building	Location
Related documentation	

3. Assessment			
Is oxygen deficiency a factor?	yes	no	
What contaminants are present?			
In what form are the contaminants?	particulate	gas/vapour	mixed
Minimum protection factor required	high	medium	low
Duration of operation			
Physical work rate	high	medium	low
Are extremes of temperature likely to be present?	yes	no	
Mobility required	normal	abnormal	
Visibility required	normal	abnormal	
Communication system required	yes	no	
Other PPE which may interfere with RPE			
Have instructions been prepared to cover foreseeable hazards associated with the use of the equipment?	yes	no	
Final choice of equipment	Maximum duration of use		
Filter type (if applicable)			

4.   General comments

5.   Date of assessment

Signatures	Date

Further reading

Croner's Risk Assessment. Croner Publications Ltd, Kingston-upon-Thames.

Croner's COSHH in Practice. Croner Publications Ltd, Kingston-upon-Thames.

Health and Safety Executive (1977) *Rationalization of Risk Assessment and Other Common Provisions in Health and Safety Legislation*. HSE Books, Sudbury, Suffolk.

Health and Safety Executive (1979) *Hot Work, Welding and Cutting on Plant Containing Flammable Materials HS(G)*. HSE Books, Sudbury, Suffolk.

Health and Safety Executive (1985) *Cleaning and Gas Freeing of Tanks Containing Flammable Residues CS5*. HSE Books, Sudbury, Suffolk.

Health and Safety Executive (1986) *Keeping LPG in Cylinders and Similar Containers CSE*. HSE Books, Sudbury, Suffolk.

Health and Safety Executive (1987) *First Aid at Work: General Guidelines for Inclusion in First Aid Boxes IND(G) 4*. HSE Books, Sudbury, Suffolk.

Health and Safety Executive (1987) *Programmable Electronic Systems: An Introductory Guide*. HSE Books, Sudbury, Suffolk.

Health and Safety Executive (1987) *Programmable Electronic Systems: General Guidelines*. HSE Books, Sudbury, Suffolk.

Health and Safety Executive (1989) *A Guide to the Pressure Systems and Transportable Gas Containers Regulations 1989 HS(R)30*. HSE Books, Sudbury, Suffolk.

Health and Safety Executive (1989) *Memorandum of Guidance on the Electricity at Work Regulations 1989 HS(R)30*. HSE Books, Sudbury, Suffolk.

Health and Safety Executive (1989) *Writing Your Health and Safety Policy Statement: Preparing a Safety Policy Statement for a Small Business*. HSE Books, Sudbury, Suffolk.

Health and Safety Executive (1990) *Dangerous Substances on Site: Notification and Warning IND(G)92(L)*. HSE Books, Sudbury, Suffolk.

Health and Safety Executive (1990) *First Aid at Work Health and Safety (First Aid) Regulations 1981. Approved Code of Practice COP42*. HSE Books, Sudbury, Suffolk.

Health and Safety Executive (1990) *A Guide to the Notification and Marking of Sites in Accordance with the Dangerous Substances (Notification and Marking of Sites) Regulations 1990 HSR29*. HSE Books, Sudbury, Suffolk.

Health and Safety Executive (1990) *The Safe Use of Portable Electrical Apparatus PM32*. HSE Books, Sudbury, Suffolk.

Health and Safety Executive (1990) *The Storage of Flammable Liquids in Fixed Tanks (up to 10,000 m^3 total capacity) HSG50*. HSE Books, Sudbury, Suffolk.

Health and Safety Executive (1991) *Assessment of Fire Hazards from Solid Materials and the Precautions Required for their Safe Storage and Use: A Guide for Manufacturers, Suppliers, Storekeepers and Users HSG64*. HSE Books, Sudbury, Suffolk.

Health and Safety Executive (1991) *The Storage of Flammable Liquids in Fixed Tanks (exceeding 10,000 m^3 total capacity) HSG52*. HSE Books, Sudbury, Suffolk.

Health and Safety Executive (1992) *Chemical Manufacturing: Permit-to-work Systems IND(G)98L*. HSE Books, Sudbury, Suffolk.

Health and Safety Executive (1992) *Dangerous Maintenance: A Study of Maintenance Accidents and How to Prevent Them*. HSE Books, Sudbury, Suffolk.

Health and Safety Executive (1992) *Five Steps to Successful Health and Safety: Special Help for Directors and Managers IND(G)132L*. HSE Books, Sudbury, Suffolk.

Health and Safety Executive (1992) *The Management of Health and Safety at Work Regulations Approved Code of Practice L21*. HSE Books, Sudbury, Suffolk.

Health and Safety Executive (1992) *Storage of Packed Dangerous Substances HSG71*. HSE Books, Sudbury, Suffolk.

Health and Safety Executive (1992) *Work Equipment: Provision and Use of Work Equipment Regulations 1992 Guidance on Regulations L22*. HSE Books, Sudbury, Suffolk.

Health and Safety Executive (1993) *Chemical Manufacturing: Prepared for EMERGENCY! IND(G)155L*. HSE Books, Sudbury, Suffolk.

Health and Safety Executive (1993) *A Step by Step Guide to COSHH Assessment HSG97*. HSE Books, Sudbury, Suffolk.

Health and Safety Executive (1994) *Electricity at Work Regulations Guidance for Small Businesses IND(G)89L*. HSE Books, Sudbury, Suffolk.

Health and Safety Executive (1994) *Five Steps to Risk Assessment IND(G)163*. HSE Books, Sudbury, Suffolk.

Health and Safety Executive (1994) *Maintaining Portable and Transportable Electrical Equipment HSG107*. HSE Books, Sudbury, Suffolk.

Health and Safety Executive (1994) *The Safe Handling of Combustible Dusts: Precautions against Explosions HSG103*. HSE Books, Sudbury, Suffolk.

Health and Safety Executive (1994) *Written Schemes of Examination Pressure Systems and Transportable Gas Containers Regulations 1989 IND(G)178L*. HSE Books, Sudbury, Suffolk.

Health and Safety Executive (1995) *CHIP 2 for Everyone HSG126*. HSE Books, Sudbury, Suffolk.

Health and Safety Executive (1995) *The Complete Idiot's Guide to CHIP 2 IND(G)181L*. HSE Books, Sudbury, Suffolk.

Health and Safety Executive (1995) *Energetic and Spontaneously Combustible Substances: Identification and Safe Handling HSG131*. HSE Books, Sudbury, Suffolk.

Health and Safety Executive (1995) *Entry into Confined Spaces GS5*. HSE Books, Sudbury, Suffolk.

Health and Safety Executive (1995) *Health Risk Management: A Practical Guide for Managers in Small and Medium Sized Enterprises HSG137*. HSE Books, Sudbury, Suffolk.

Health and Safety Executive (1995) *Out of Control: Why Control Systems go Wrong and How to Prevent Failure*. HSE Books, Sudbury, Suffolk.

Health and Safety Executive (1995) *Read the Label: How to Find Out if Chemicals are Dangerous IND(G)186L*. HSE Books, Sudbury, Suffolk.

Health and Safety Executive (1995) *Safety Data Sheets for Substances and Preparations Dangerous for Supply. Guidance on Regulation 6 of the CHIP Regulations 1994 Approved Code of Practice L62*. HSE Books, Sudbury, Suffolk.

Health and Safety Executive (1995) *Why Do I Need a Safety Data Sheet? IND(G)182L*. HSE Books, Sudbury, Suffolk.

Health and Safety Executive (1996) *Approved Carriage List: Information Approved for the Carriage of Dangerous Goods by Road and Rail Other Than Explosives and Radioactive Material L90*. HSE Books, Sudbury, Suffolk.

Health and Safety Executive (1996) *Approved Requirements for the Construction of Vehicles for the Carriage of Explosives by Road, Carriage of Explosives by Road Regulations 1996 L92*. HSE Books, Sudbury, Suffolk.

Health and Safety Executive (1996) *Approved Requirements for the Packaging, Labelling and Carriage of Radioactive Material by Rail. Packaging, Labelling and Carriage of Radioactive Material by Rail Regulation 1996 L94*. HSE Books, Sudbury, Suffolk.

Health and Safety Executive (1996) *Approved Requirements and Test Methods for the Classification and Packing of Dangerous Goods for Carriage L88*. HSE Books, Sudbury, Suffolk.

Health and Safety Executive (1996) *Approved Supply Lists, Third Edition, Information Approved for the Classification and Labelling of Substances and Preparations Dangerous for Supply Including Supplement L76*. HSE Books, Sudbury, Suffolk.

Health and Safety Executive (1996) *Approved Tank Requirements: The Provision for Bottom Loading and Vapour Recovery Systems of Mobile Containers Carrying Petrol. Carrying of Dangerous Goods by Road Regulations 1996 L93*. HSE Books, Sudbury, Suffolk.

Health and Safety Executive (1996) *Approved Vehicle Requirements Carriage of Dangerous Goods by Road Regulations 1996 L89*. HSE Books, Sudbury, Suffolk.

Health and Safety Executive (1996) *The Carriage of Dangerous Goods Explained: Part 1. Guidance for Consignors of Dangerous Goods by Rail (Classification, Packaging, Labelling and Provision for Information) HSG160*. HSE Books, Sudbury, Suffolk.

Health and Safety Executive (1996) *The Carriage of Dangerous Goods Explained: Part 2. Guidance for Road Vehicle Operators and Others Involved in the Carriage of Dangerous Goods by Road HSG161*. HSE Books, Sudbury, Suffolk.

Health and Safety Executive (1996) *The Carriage of Dangerous Goods Explained: Part 3. Guidance for Rail Operators and Others Involved in the Carriage of Dangerous Goods by Rail HSG163*. HSE Books, Sudbury, Suffolk.

Health and Safety Executive (1996) *The Carriage of Dangerous Goods Explained: Part 4. Guidance for Operators, Drivers and Others Involved in the Carriage of Explosives by Road HSG162*. HSE Books, Sudbury, Suffolk.

Health and Safety Executive (1996) *The Carriage of Dangerous Goods Explained: Part 5. Guidance for Consignors, Rail Operators, and Others Involved in the Packaging, Labelling and Carriage of Radioactive Material by Rail HSG164*. HSE Books, Sudbury, Suffolk.

Health and Safety Executive (1996) *Everyone's Guide to RIDDOR'95 HSE31*. HSE Books, Sudbury, Suffolk.

Health and Safety Executive (1996) *A Guide to Reporting of Injuries, Diseases and Dangerous Occurrences Regulations L73*. HSE Books, Sudbury, Suffolk.

Health and Safety Executive (1996) *Lift-trucks in Potentially Flammable Atmospheres HSG113*. HSE Books, Sudbury, Suffolk.

Health and Safety Executive (1996) *The Safe Use and Handling of Flammable Liquids HSG140*. HSE Books, Sudbury, Suffolk.

Health and Safety Executive (1996) *Safe Working with Flammable Substances INDG227L*. HSE Books, Sudbury, Suffolk.

Health and Safety Executive (1996) *Suitability of Vehicles and Containers and Limits on Quantities for the Carriage of Explosives, Carriage of Explosives by Road Regulations 1996 Approved Code of Practice L91*. HSE Books, Sudbury, Suffolk.

Health and Safety Executive (1997) *Emergency Action for Burns IND(G)161L*. HSE Books, Sudbury, Suffolk.

Health and Safety Executive (1997) *First Aid at Work: Your Questions Answered INDF214*. HSE Books, Sudbury, Suffolk.

Health and Safety Executive (1997) *Guidance on Permit-to-work in the Petroleum Industry*. HSE Books, Sudbury, Suffolk.

Health and Safety Executive (1997) *Managing Contractors: A Guide for Employers*. HSE Books, Sudbury, Suffolk.

Health and Safety Executive (1997) *Safety Signs and Signals: The Health and Safety (Safety Signs and Signals) Regulations 1996*. HSE Books, Sudbury, Suffolk.

Health and Safety Executive (1997) *Successful Health and Safety Management HSG65*. HSE Books, Sudbury, Suffolk.

Health and Safety Executive (1998) *The Storage of Flammable Liquids in Containers HSG51*. HSE Books, Sudbury, Suffolk.

HSC 6 *Writing a Safety Policy Statement: Advice to Employees.*

Kluwer's Handbook of Risk Management. Croner Publications Ltd, Kingston-upon-Thames.

Principles of Health and Safety and Work. Institute of Occupational Safety and Health, Leicester.

SI (1972) SI 1972/917 *The Highly Flammable Liquids and Liquefied Petroleum Gases Regulations*. HMSO, London.

SI (1976) SI 1976/2003 *The Health and Safety (Etc.) Act 1974*. HMSO, London.

SI (1977) SI 1977/500 *The Safety Representative and Safety Committee Regulations*. HMSO, London.

SI (1981) SI 1981/917 *The Control of Lead at Work Regulations 1980*. HMSO, London.

SI (1989) SI 1989/1790 *The Noise at Work Regulations 1989*. HMSO, London.

SI (1989) SI 1989/2169 *The Pressure Systems and Transportable Gas Containers Regulations 1989*. HMSO, London.

SI (1990) SI 1990/304 *Dangerous Substances (Notification and Marking of Sites) Regulations 1990*. HMSO, London.

SI (1992) SI 1992/2051 *The Management of Health and Safety at Work Regulations 1992*. HMSO, London.

SI (1992) SI 1992/2793 *The Manual Handling Operations Regulations 1992*. HMSO, London.

SI (1992) *The Personal Protective Equipment at Work Regulations 1992*. HMSO, London.

SI (1992) SI 1992/2932 *The Provision and Use of Work Equipment Regulations 1992*. HMSO, London.

SI (1992) SI 1992/3004 *The Workplace (Health, Safety and Welfare) Regulations 1992*. HMSO, London.

SI (1994) SI 1994/1746 *The Chemicals (Hazard Information and Packaging for Supply) Regulations 1994*. HMSO, London.

SI (1994) SI 1994/3246 *The Control of Substances Hazardous to Health Regulations 1994*. HMSO, London.

SI (1995) SI 1995 *The Reporting of Injuries, Diseases and Dangerous Occurrences Regulations 1995*. HMSO, London.

SI (1996) SI 1996/2092 *The Carriage of Dangerous Goods (Classification, Packaging and Labelling) and Use of Transportable Pressure Receptacles Regulations 1996*. HMSO, London.

SI (1996) SI 1996/2089 *The Carriage of Dangerous Goods by Rail Regulations 1996*. HMSO, London.

SI (1996) SI 1996/2094 *The Carriage of Dangerous Goods by Road (Driver Training) Regulations 1996*. HMSO, London.

SI (1996) SI 1996/2095 *The Carriage of Dangerous Goods by Road Regulations 1996*. HMSO, London.

SI (1996) SI 1996/2093 *The Carriage of Explosives by Road Regulations 1996*. HMSO, London.

SI (1996) SI 1996/192 *The Equipment and Protective Systems Intended for Use in Potentially Explosive Atmospheres Regulations 1996*. HMSO, London.

SI (1996) SI 1996/1513 *The Health and Safety (Consultation with Employees) Regulations 1996*. HMSO, London.

SI (1996) SI 1996/341 *The Health and Safety (Safety Signs and Signals) Regulations 1996*. HMSO, London.

SI (1996) SI 1996/2075 *The Health and Safety at Work (Etc.) Act 1974 (Application to Environmentally Hazardous Substances) Regulations 1996*. HMSO, London.

SI (1996) SI 1996/2090 *The Packing, Labelling and Carriage of Radioactive Material by Rail Regulations 1996*. HMSO, London.

The Control of Asbestos at Work Regulations 1987. HMSO, London.

The Electricity at Work Regulations 1989. HMSO, London.

The Factories Act 1961. HMSO, London.

The Fire Certificate (Special Premises) Regulations. HMSO, London.

The Fire Precautions Act, 1971 (enforced by the Fire Authority). HMSO, London.

The Health and Safety (First Aid) Regulations 1981. HMSO, London.

The Petroleum Consolidation Act 1928. HMSO, London.

Appendix I: Suppliers of equipment

Acoustic calibrators: *see* Sound level meters
Adsorbent tubes: Casella, Negretti Automation, Perkin Elmer
Anemometers and air flow meters: Airflow Developments, ATP, Biral,
  British Rototherm, Casella, EIM, Prosser Scientific Instruments, Testo
Balances: Mettler-Toledo, Sanyo Gallenkamp, Sartorius Instruments
Bubblers (impingers): Casella, JS Holdings, Sanyo Gallenkamp, SKC
Carrying cases: Delsey, Topper Cases
Colorimetric gas detectors: Anachem, Drager, Protector Technologies
Diaphragm pressure gauges: Control Centre
Direct reading dust instruments: Biral, Casella, Gelman Sciences, MDA,
  Negretti Automation
Direct reading gas instruments: Crowcon, Casella, Drager, HNU Systems,
  MDA, MSA, Morganite, Negretti Automation, Protector Technologies,
  Quantitech, Shaw City, Zellweger
Dust lamps: Cluson Engineering
Filter holders: AC, Casella, EIM, Gelman Sciences, Negretti Automation,
  SKC
Filters (air sampling): Gelman Sciences, JS Holdings, Millipore, Sanyo
  Gallenkamp, Sartorius, Whatman
Flow meters and calibrators: Casella, EIM, JS Holdings, Platon, SKC
Forceps: Sanyo Gallenkamp
General electrical equipment: Radio Spares
General laboratory equipment: Sanyo Gallenkamp
Harnesses: Casella, Negretti Automation
Heat stress monitors: Casella, Metrosonics, Shaw City
Hire companies: Livingstone Rental,
Kata thermometers: Casella, Charnwood
Light meters: *see* photometers
Manometers: Airflow Developments
Microbiological samplers: Abinghurst Biotest, Casella, Gelman Sciences,
  Millipore, Sartorius
Microscope dispersion staining objective: McCrone Scientific
Microscope eyepiece graticules: Graticules
Microscope slide mounting fluids: McCrone Scientific
Microscope slides and cover glasses: Sanyo Gallenkamp
Microscopes: Carl Zeiss, Gallenkamp, Leica Microsystems
Microwave meter: Rohde and Schwarz
Noise dosimeters: Bruel and Kjaer, Castle Group, CEL, Cirrus, Reten, Shaw
  City, PC Werth
Optical particle counters: Gelman Sciences
Paper tape detectors: MDA
Passive samplers: Casella, Drager, 3M, Perkin Elmer, Shaw City, SKC
Photocells: Diffusion Systems Ltd
Photometers: Able, ATP, EIM, Hagner, R & S Components
Pistonphones: Bruel and Kjaer
Pitot-static tubes: Airflow Developments, Casella
Pressure gauges: Airflow Developments, Control Centre
Psychrometers (hygrometers): Airflow Developments, Casella
Psychrometric charts: CIBSE

Pumps (air sampling): AC, Biral, Casella Ltd, EIM, Gillian, JS Holdings, MDA, Negretti Automation, Pascal Scientific, Shaw City, Sypol

Radiation monitors: Amersham International, Casella, Cherwell Laboratories, Difco, GEC, Lablogic Systems, KCI, Lab M, Mini Instruments, Negretti, NRPB, NE Technology, Siemens, Southern Scientific, Wardray Products

Rotameters: Casella, EIM, Pascal Scientific, Platon, Sanyo Gallenkamp, SKC

Sampling bags: Casella, SKC

Smoke tubes: Airflow Developments, Drager,

Sound level meters: Bruel and Kjaer, Castle Group, CEL, Cirrus, EIM, Reten, Shaw City, PC Werth

Thermal environment meters: Bruel and Kjaer, Casella, Shaw City

Thermometers: Casella, Charnwood Instrumentation, Comark, Sanyo Gallenkamp

Tracer gas krypton Kr85: Amersham International

Tubing (laboratory): *red/blue plastic*, Airflow Developments; *clear*, Sanyo Gallenkamp

Wind tunnel (open jet): Airflow Developments

Appendix II: Addresses of suppliers

Abinghurst Ltd, Unit 1, Ross Road Business Centre, Northampton, NN5 5AX, tel: 01604 581111

Able Instruments and Controls Ltd, Cutbush Park, Danehill, Lower Earley, Reading, Berks, RG6 4UT, tel: 01734 311188

Airflow Developments Ltd, Lancaster Road, Cressex Business Park, High Wycombe, Bucks, HP12 3QP, tel: 01494 525252

Amersham International Plc, Amersham Place, Little Chalfont, Amersham, Bucks, HP7 9NA, tel: 01494 544000

Anachem Ltd, 20 Charles Street, Luton, Beds, LU2 OEB, tel: 01582 745000

AC Technical Safety, Beeston House, Princess Gardens, Newport, Shropshire, TF10 7ET, tel: 01952 820155

Autonic Research Ltd, Tollesbury, Essex, CM9 8SE, tel: 01621 869460

Biral, Bristol Industrial and Research Associates Ltd, PO Box 2, Portishead, Bristol, BS20 9JB, tel: 01275 847787

British Rototherm Company Ltd, Kenfig Industrial Estate, Margam, Port Talbot, West Glam, SA13 2PW, tel: 01656 740551

Bruel and Kjaer (UK) Ltd, Harrow Weald Lodge, 92 Uxbridge Road, Harrow, Middlesex, HA3 6BZ, tel: 0181 954 2366

Carl Zeiss Ltd, PO Box 78, 17–20 Woodfield Road, Welwyn Garden City, Herts, AL7 1LU, tel: 01707 331144

Casella Ltd, Regent House, Kempston, Bedford, MK42 7JY, tel: 01234 841441

Castle Group Ltd, Salter Road, Cayton Low Road Industrial Estate, Scarborough, N. Yorks, YO11 3UZ, tel: 01723 584250

CEL Instruments, 35–37 Bury Mead Road, Hitchin, Herts, SG5 1RT, tel: 01462 422411

Charnwood Instrumentation Services, 81 Park Road, Coalville, Leics, LE67 3AF, tel: 01530 510615

Cherwell Laboratories, 114 Churchill Road, Bicester, Oxon, OX6 7XB, tel: 01869 241911

CIBSE, Chartered Institute of Building Services Engineers, 222 Balham High Road, London SW12 9BS, tel: 0181 675 5211

Cirrus Research Ltd, Acoustic House, Bridlington Road, Hunmanby, N. Yorks, YO14 0PH, tel: 01723 891655

Cluson Engineering Ltd, Unit 6, Bedford Road, Petersfield, Hants, GU32 3LJ, tel: 01730 264672

Comark Ltd, Swallowfield, Welwyn Garden City, Herts, AL7 1JP, tel: 01707 331051

Control Centre, 63 Pritchetts Street, Birmingham, B6 4EX, tel: 0121 359 8207

Crowcon Detection Instruments Ltd, 2 Blacklands Way, Abingdon Business Park, Abingdon, Oxon, OX14 1DY, tel: 01235 553057

Dawe Instruments (*see* CEL Instruments)

Delsey, large retail stores

Difco, PO Box 14B, Central Avenue, West Molesley, Surrey, KT8 2SE, tel: 0181 979 9951

Diffusion Systems Ltd, 43 Rosebank Road, London NW7 2EW, tel: 0181 579 5231

Draeger Limited, Ullswater Close, Kitty Brewster Industrial Estate, Blyth, Northumberland, NE24 4RG, tel: 01670 352891

EIM, Environmental and Industrial Monitoring, 11 Stokes Lane, Haddenham, Bucks, HP17 8DY, tel: 01844 290624

GEC Alsthon Engineering Systems Ltd, Cambridge Road, Whetstone, Leics, LE8 6LH, tel: 0116 275 0750

Gallenkamp (*see* Sanyo Gallenkamp)

Gelman Sciences, Brackmills Business Park, Caswell Road, Northampton, NN4 7EZ, tel: 01604 765141

Graticules Ltd, Fircrost Way, Edenbridge, Kent, TN8 6HA, tel: 01732 864863

Hagner Photometric Instruments Ltd, Brooks Lane, Bosham, Chichester, Sussex, tel: 01243 575723

Haden Laboratories, Haden House, Chiltern Hill, Chalfont St Peter, Bucks, SL9 9UG, tel: 01753 888447

HNU Systems Ltd, 15 Tanning Court, Howley, Warrington, Lancs, WA1 2HF, tel: 01925 445941

JS Holdings, Unit 5, Willows Link, Stevenage, Herts, SG2 8AB, tel: 01438 316994

KCI Medical Ltd, Wareham, Dorset, BH20 4SP, tel: 01929 556 576

Lablogic Systems Ltd, St Johns House, 131 Psalter Lane, Sheffield, S11 8UX, tel: 0114 250 0419

Lab M, Topley House, 52 Wash Lane, Bury, Lancs, BL9 6AU, tel: 0161 797 5729

Larson Davis Ltd, Redcar Station Business Centre, Station Road, Redcar, Cleveland, TS10 2RD, tel: 01642 491565

Leica Micro Systems, Davy Avenue, Knowle Hill, Milton Keynes, MK5 8LB, tel: 01908 666663

Leitz (*see* Leica Micro Systems)

Livingstone Rental, 2 Queens Road, Teddington, Middlesex, TW11 0LB, tel: 0800 886000

3M United Kingdom Plc, 28 Great Jackson Street, Manchester, M15 4PA, tel: 0161 236 8500

McCrone Scientific Ltd, McCrone House, 155A Leighton Road, London, NW5 2RD, tel: 0171 267 7199

MDA Scientific (UK) Ltd, Unit 10, Boleyn Court, Manor Park, Runcorn, WA7 1SR, tel: 01928 579224

Mettler-Toledo Ltd, 64 Boston Road, Beaumont Leys, Leicester, LE4 1AW

Millipore (UK) Ltd, The Boulevard, Blackmore Lane, Watford, Herts, WD1 8YW, tel: 01923 816375

Mini Instruments Ltd, 15 Burnham Business Park, Springfield Road, Burnham-on-Crouch, Essex, CM0 8TE, tel: 01621 783282

Morganite Electronic Instruments Ltd (*see* Mini Instruments Ltd)

MSA (Britain) Ltd, East Shawhead, Coatbridge, Midlothian, ML5 4TD, tel: 01236 424966

Negretti Automation Ltd, Aylesbury Industrial Centre, Bicester Road, Aylesbury, Bucks, HP19 3AL, tel: 01296 395931

Neotronics (*see* Zellweger Analytics Ltd)

NRPB, National Radiological Protection Board Dosimetry Service, Chilton, Didcot, Oxon, OX11 0GQ, tel: 01235 834590

NE Technology Ltd, Bath Road, Beenham, Reading, RG7 5PR, tel: 0118 971 2121

Pascal Scientific Ltd, 10 Chesterfield Way, Pump Lane, Hayes, Middlesex, UB3 3NW

Perkin Elmer Ltd, Post Office Lane, Beaconsfield, Bucks, HP9 1QA, tel: 01494 676161

Platon Instrumentation Ltd, Platon Park, Viables, Basingstoke, RG22 4BS, tel: 01256 470456

Plessey Controls (*see* Siemens)

Prosser Scientific Instruments, Lady Lane Industrial Estate, Hadleigh, Suffolk, IP7 6BQ, tel: 01473 823005

Protector Technologies Group, Ash Road, Aldershot, Hants, GU12 4DE, tel: 01252 342352

Quantitech Ltd, Unit 3 Old Wolverton Road, Old Wolverton, Milton Keynes, Bucks, MK12 5NP, tel: 01908 227722

R & S Components, PO Box 99, Birchington Road, Corby, NN17 9RS, tel: 01536 201201

Raytest Instruments (*see* Lablogic Systems Ltd)

Reten Acoustics, Ty Coch House, Llantarnam Park Way, Cwmbran, Gwent, NP44 3AW, tel: 01633 877855

Rohde and Schwarz (UK) Ltd, Ancells Business Park, Fleet, Hants, GU13 8UZ, tel: 01252 811377

Royco (see Gelman)

Sabre Gas Detection (*see* Protector Technologies)

Salford Electrical Instruments Ltd, Peel Works, Barton Lane, Eccles, Manchester, M30 0HL, tel: 0161 839 5900

Sanyo Gallenkamp Plc, 50 Bishop Meadow Road, Loughborough, Leics, LE11 0RE, tel: 01509 265265

Sartorius Instruments Ltd, Longmead Business Centre, Blenheim Road, Epsom, Surrey, KT19 9QN, tel: 01372 745811

Siemens, Sopers Lane, Poole, Dorset, BH17 7ER, tel: 01202 782000

Shaw City Ltd, Pioneer Road, Faringdon, Oxon, SN7 7BU, tel: 01367 241675

SKC Ltd, Unit 11, Sunrise Park, Blandford Forum, Dorset, DT11 8ST, tel: 01258 480188

Southern Scientific Ltd, Scientific House, Rectory Farm Road, Sompting, Lancing, Sussex, BN15 0DP, tel: 01903 604000

R.A. Stephen & Co. Ltd, 8 Station Road Industrial Estate, Burnham-on-Crouch, CM0 8RN, tel: 01621 783282

Sypol, Market House, Market Square, Aylesbury, Bucks, HP20 1TN, tel: 01296 415715

Testo Ltd, 3 Oriel Court, Omega Park, Alton, Hampshire, GU34 2QE, tel: 01420 544433

3M (UK) Plc, 3M House, PO Box 1, Bracknell, RG12 1JU, tel: 01344 858000

Topper Cases, St Peters Hill, Huntingdon, Cambs, PE18 7DX, tel: 01480 457251

Vickers Instruments, Haxby Road, York, YO3 7SD, tel: 01904 631351

Wardray Products Ltd, Hampton Court Estate, Summer Road, Thames Ditton, KT7 0SP, tel: 0181 398 9911

P.C. Werth Ltd, Audiology House, 45 Nightingale Lane, London SW12 8SP, tel: 0181 675 5151

Whatman Laboratory Products, Springfield Mill, Maidstone, ME14 2LE, tel: 01622 692022

Zellweger Analytics Ltd, Parsonage Road, Takeley, Bishops Stortford, Herts, CM22 6PU, tel: 01279 870182

Index